Case Studies on Practice Development

edited by
James Dooher, Andrew Clark and
John Fowler

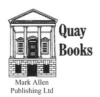

Quay
Books

Mark Allen
Publishing Ltd

Quay Books Division, Mark Allen Publishing Ltd
Jesses Farm, Snow Hill, Dinton, Nr Salisbury, Wiltshire, SP3 5HN

British Library Cataloguing-in-Publication Data
A catalogue record is available for this book

© Mark Allen Publishing Ltd 2001

ISBN 1 85642 169 4

Printed in the UK by The Cromwell Press, Trowbridge, Wiltshire

Contents

Acknowledgements

Our grateful thanks go to all contributors who despite busy lives managed to find space and time to contribute to this book. They include:

Lee Beresford RMN, M Med Sci is currently seconded to the NHS Executive Northern and Yorkshire region.

Sarah Holland Dip HE Mental Health, D Grade Staff Nurse, Regional Forensic Service.

Shams Uddin is a D Grade Staff Nurse working in acute mental health.

Sonia Maisey EN(M) Dip HE works as a D Grade Staff Nurse in a city general hospital intensive therapy unit.

Kate Diamond RGN, RM, BSc (Hons), DPSN qualified as a Registered Midwife and took up a post as a staff midwife.

Dawn Holding RMN, RGN, BA (Hons) ENB Higher Award is the Team Leader of a Mental Health Community Rehabilitation Team (CRT).

Penny Harrison RGN, BA (Hons), ENB 100 Cert Ed was the Clinical Team Leader (CTL) for the Gastroenterology Process at the Leicester Royal Infirmary.

Gordon Gadsby PhD, BA(Hons), RGN, RMN, DipN (Lond) MISBM, DHP, DHS, is a Nurse Practitioner/Lecturer in complementary therapies.

June Freehan RGN, RHV, RM, BA (Hons), ENB Higher Award is a Health Visitor.

Bernice Litchfield RGN is a Nurse Endoscopist within the gastro-intestinal department of a large city hospital.

Alison Wells RGN, RM Dip N, Dip Ed, BA (Hons) currently works as change manager within a centre of best practice in a large city hospital.

Adrian Hastings MB Ch B is a Teaching Co-ordinator at the Department of General Practice and Primary Health Care, University of Leicester and a partner in a busy GP practice.

Jonathan Carver RGN, BSc (Hons), ENB Higher Award, ENB 124, Cert Health Ed works as a Lecturer Practitioner specialising in cardiac nursing.

Sally Rudge RMN, RNMH, BA(Hons), Dip Psy, ACBS, MSc is a community nurse working for adults with a learning disability.

Helen Jones BSc, RGN, Cert Ed (FE), RNT, MA works in a large teaching hospital as a Senior Nurse Research and Development Officer.

Chris Hale RGN, PN Cert, Moorlands Cert, ITEC has an advisory and facilitative role for nurses working within general practice settings.

Frazer Underwood RGN, Dip HE Nursing worked as a key worker on an acute stroke unit .

Sandra Kemp RGN, RSCN is a Clinical Team Leader in respiratory paediatrics in the Children's Hospital at the Leicester Royal Infirmary.

Jim Bailey SRN, RMN, BSc (Hons) Psychol RNT, Cert Ed (FE), Cert Dynamic Psy, Registered UKCP is a Principal Psychotherapist within the NHS.

Rachel North RGN, RHV, DPSN, BA (Hons) is a Directorate Nurse Advisor.

Dr Deenesh Khoosal LLM(RCS), LLM(RCP)–(Ire), BAO, MB, BCh, FRC Psych works as Consultant Psychiatrist, Clinical Tutor, and also as an Examiner for the Royal College of Psychiatrists.

Dean Hart RMN is a Day Hospital Manager and Practice Development Nurse.

Preface

The world of health care practice contains numerous examples of 'ordinary' practitioners developing innovative and creative ideas as part of their daily work. A number of practice developments arise from small scale projects that were developed to meet a specific need in a particular environment. One of the areas that many of the health care professions are currently grappling with is the development of a culture which enables the validation of practise-based research, thus enhancing the development of theoretical models out of practice rather than the traditional application of theory to practice. One of the ways of engaging in this process is to reflect upon critical and innovative practices and discuss them with others.

This book contains a number of reflective accounts from a range of health care practitioners. The contributors were asked to describe and reflect upon a challenging and innovative aspect of their role that was meaningful to them at their particular point in their career. The editors imposed no single model of reflection on the contributors as it was felt that this would lead to an artificial and restrictive style for many contributors.

Within this book you will find a number of interesting approaches to practice development. The focus of some of the illustrations are specific to the speciality, eg. the endoscopy specialist, for others the focus is more generic. However even if you as the reader do not relate to the clinical speciality, you should be able to relate to the more fundamental principles of how practice is being developed or the problems that might be encountered if similar developments were undertaken. As editors we hope that you find this book not only interesting, but one that provokes questions and ideas in your mind and clinical practice.

This book begins to develop theoretical ideas from everyday practice — a bottom up approach to theory development. As a companion to this the editors have also produced *The Handbook Of Practice Development* (2001) which explores a number of theoretical ideas and their application to practice — a top down approach to theory development. Used together these complementary texts will give readers a comprehensive understanding of contemporary practice development, the challenges, shortfalls and successes of this complex concept.

About the editors

James Dooher RMN, FHE Cert Ed, Dip HCR, MA Senior Lecturer, De Montfort University, Leicester

James has worked in a variety of psychiatric settings and spent three years as a practice development nurse specialising in rehabilitation nursing before moving full time to education. He has an interest in research, practice development and is currently registered for a PhD. He is a full-time senior lecturer at De Montfort University School of Nursing and Midwifery.He is also the joint editor of *The Handbook of Practice Development* and was a contributor to *The Handbook of Clinical Supervision – Your questions answered.*

Andrew Clark, RMN, RGN, Cpn Cert, ENB 955, FETC, DMS, MBA Part Time Lecturer/freelance educator and clinical nurse

Andrew has a wide range of experience both in patient and community-based settings and has held clinical, managerial and professional posts. Previous roles within a health care setting include Community Psychiatric Nurse, Clinical Nurse Manager, Patient Services Manager and Practice Development Nurse. He currently works independently in a clinical, consultative and training capacity in both the private and public education sectors. He is also the joint editor of *The Handbook of Practice Development* and was a contributor for *The Handbook of Clinical Supervision – Your questions answered.*

John Fowler, RGN, RMN, RCNT, RNT, Dip N, Cert Ed, BA, MA Principal Lecturer, De Montfort University, Leicester

John has a varied background of nursing and nurse education. He is currently programme leader for the Health Care Practice Programme at DeMontfort University. This encompasses a variety of post registration ENB Awards and the UKCC Specialist Practitioner Qualification. He has a particular interest in clinical supervision and the development of practice. He is also the joint editor of *The Handbook of Practice Development* and was the editor for *The Handbook of Clinical Supervision – Your questions answered.*

How to use this book

As the companion to *The Handbook of Practice Development* (Clark, Dooher and Fowler, 2001) this book explores accounts and examples of individuals' reflections on their own practice development.

The book will give the reader an insight into the reflections of others and will hopefully inspire you in turn, to reflect upon your own professional experiences. It is not a book aimed at teaching you how you should engage in the reflective process. Indeed, the editors have deliberately steered away from that path including only a brief introduction to reflection, in order that you may judge for yourselves the merits and style of each reflection and choose your own way forward. You will find in the reference section additional reading material to assist you in your choice of reflective model.

Contributions are presented from clinicians, team leaders independent practitioners/lecturers, practitioners/strategic policy makers from many areas of health care. The ability to reflect is not synonymous either with seniority in an organisational sense nor level of clinical expertise, and it is a valuable exercise for everyone.

You may wish to start at page one and read sequentially. However each reflection stands alone so you may choose if you wish to dip into single reflections.

The book is constructed in a way which takes the reader on a journey through early reflective accounts from student nurses to clinical-based experiences and strategic interpretations of practice development. It is important to understand that a professional's grade, rank or ascribed level of responsibility, does not necessarily mean that they are any less or more skilled at the reflective process.

Each of the reflective accounts is preceded with a short summary and followed with annotations from the editors with key questions and discussion points for the reader.

The views expressed by the individual contributors are not necessarily those of the editors. All contributions have been peer-reviewed and all patient names been altered to protect each individual's identity.

Enjoy reflecting on the reflections of others. Remember practice development is the responsibility of each and every individual practitioner.

The reflective practice cycle (adapted from Gibbs *et al*, 1988)

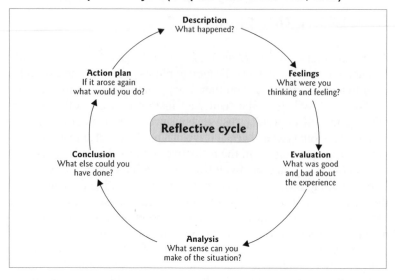

Introduction: reflection — an overview

Lee Beresford and Andrew Clark

Reflection is a very personal thing, like clinical supervision there is no one model that will meet everyone's requirements. You must try different methods and models to find the one that suits you. It is important to remember that reflection is a means to an end and not an end in itself.

Reflective practice is a common feature in the nursing literature and to a greater or lesser extent is now an accepted part of nursing practice development. It is frequently referred to though often ill defined, which in part is due to the inadequate conceptualisation of the process of reflection (James and Clark, 1994). There have been many attempts to define reflective practice but some authors such as Atkins, Murphy and Goff (1993) argue that the concept is poorly defined.

Additionally, although many nurses have come to understand the need to reflect on their practice, reflection does not simply occur as a result of knowing about it (Wilkinson, 1999). However, the requirement for post registered nurses to maintain a personal profile effectively means that they are obliged to engage in some reflective activity (Andrews, Gidman and Humphreys, 1998). It is doubtful however whether most nurses have experience of facilitation to assist them with the process.

Nearly seventy years ago, educationalist and thinker Dewey (1933) reasoned that the origins of all thinking lay in the encounter of problematic situations. These could be defined as situations that cannot be resolved through the employment of prior solutions. Dewey strongly emphasised the active nature of learning, and argued that learning is not achieved by experience alone, rather that thought and consideration (reflection) are, in addition to experience, integral to the process of learning. For those studying reflection Powell's (1991) account of the history and development of reflection is highly recommended. In this excellent discourse Powell details the complex links between the origins of reflective activity and experiential learning.

In the early 1970s, some scholars and, in particular Habermas (1971), began to further develop the concept of reflection, and to formulate notions of 'critical intent' as a quality with which people would enter reflective activity. Twelve years later, building upon the work of Habermas, Mezirow (1983) postulated a new concept of a hierarchy of reflective activity modelled on seven progressive levels. An attempt to map out Mezirow's hierarchy is illustrated in *Figure Introduction.1.*

Figure Introduction.1: Mezirow's hierarchy

R	**Reflectivity** Awareness of specific perceptions, thoughts, actions, behaviours and meanings	
E	**Affective reflectivity** Awareness of feelings that are associated with the perception	*Awareness*
F	**Discriminant reflectivity** Awareness of the effectiveness of perceptions	
L	**Judgemental reflectivity** Awareness of value judgements regarding perceptions	
E	**Conceptual reflectivity** Consciousness of the awareness and questioning of the perception	
C	**Psychic reflectivity** Judgements are made on perceived evidence which is constrained by the experience and awareness of the perceiver	*Critical thought*
T	**Theoretical reflectivity** Better judgements may be made by altering perspectives	

In constructing his hierarchy, Mezirow defines a boundary between a simple state of awareness in the reflector, and where critical thought is in active use. For Mezirow it is beyond this boundary that perceptions are transformed. An alternative way of viewing and understanding Mezirow's work is suggested by Powell (1991) who offers the concept of a continuum beginning with reflective activity and ending with altered perspectives.

This stance is complemented by Boyd and Fales (1983) who explored ideas about reflection in the learning process. This learning process is described by the authors as creating and clarifying the meaning of past or current experience in terms of an internal (spiritual) and external (worldly) self.

They also suggest that an outcome of the process is a perspective that is in some way altered. Thus, they postulate that the importance of reflective activity for health and social care professionals can be demonstrated in their growth, and the growth of those in their care. Yet, not all authors hold complementary positions to Mezirow's view. A striking example of this can be found in Kolb's (1984) work. Here reflections and actions are described as entirely distinct, quasi-antagonistic activities.

Kemmis (1985) conceptually divided reflection into three separate classes simultaneously existing in parallel to each other. They are:

* problem solving
* practical deliberation
* speculative thought.

The most interesting aspect of Kemmis' work is, however, not his basic model for understanding reflection. In 1985 Kemmis was proactive in placing more emphasis on the need to interpret reflection as a social rather than individual process.

In the same year, Boud, Keogh and Walker (1985) who were interested in developing reflection and experiential learning within broadly educative processes, talked about reflection as having two centres. These were cognitive and emotional centres, and were suggested as activities in which individuals engage to explore experiences (their own and other's) in order to lead to new or altered understanding.

Reflection in action

The concept of reflection in action has most notably been developed by Schön (1983), building on earlier work by Schön and Argyris (1974, 1978). In this seminal text, conventional academic knowledge is referred to as 'technical rationality'; and areas of professional practice are referred to as 'high hard ground' where practitioners can make effective use of research-based theory and technique. However, Schön (1983) recognises that practitioners do not deal with soluble problems through reference to this 'high hard ground'. There are other areas of professional practice where the situations they encounter are complex, indeterminate and incapable of technical solution. Schön (1983) believes these are best described as 'swampy lowlands', saying:

> *The difficulty is that the problems of the high ground, however great their technical interest, are often relatively unimportant*

to patients or to the larger society, while in the swamp are the
problems of greatest human concern.

Now the concept of reflection has been accepted, there are writers who would argue that there are dilemmas involved in the reflective process and advise caution. Burnard (1995) questions whether it is morally and ethically right to ask people to reflect on their intimate values inviting you to consider in what other profession you are asked to reveal your deepest thoughts.

There are potentially two problems. Firstly, the fear and risk of making the professionals deal with the past and not seeing the here and now, and subsequently inhibiting forward thinking looking towards the future. Secondly, perhaps there is a tendency to be selective and choose safe episodes in education and practice at a superficial level.

It is generally accepted that nurses who engage in reflective activity do so to develop their practice. However, there is little empirical evidence to suggest that practice development or improved patient care occurs as a direct result of reflection (Andrews *et al* 1998). Although this view is not held by all, it is wise to review the criticisms of reflection carefully on the grounds that because these views may be unpopular and swim against the tide, it does not necessarily mean that they are wrong.

Hargreaves (1997) argues that there are questions of ownership of knowledge to be addressed, along with the responsibilities of those professionals with this knowledge. As reflective practice often involves practitioners' subjective description and interpretation of events, these will usually include details of clients. It is debatable whether it is usual for clients to be aware of this. While one can argue that case conference discussion and so on add directly to patient care improvement, the evidence is scant which demonstrates the extent to which reflective practice equals value added. Hargreaves goes on to state that reflective practice is not simply re-examining someone's case; rather it involves personal interpretation and judgement. The reflector may be recording incidents, verbally or in written form, which otherwise may not be recorded and may be controversial.

Reflective practice differs in that value judgements are added retrospectively and there is little in the literature which questions the moral implications for patients; nor is there a great deal written about whether we should reflect, as there is a potential for vulnerability in the reflector, an aspect that is under researched. Some authors, notably Hullat (1995), go so far as to suggest that there are sometimes good reasons for not reflecting on certain events and warns of harmful consequences for those individuals who are pressurised to do so.

The future

Whatever your own personal view of reflection, it is now an established concept and nurses need to both understand it and engage in reflective activity as part of their ongoing professional development.

Perhaps the best way forward here is for the facilitator to give an example of the appropriate depth of reflection that will achieve the desired educational outcomes. This then enables the participants to choose freely the nature of their contribution and the manner in which they present it (Hullett, 1995). This should enable the vulnerability issue to be controlled.

After all, if within a responsible and ethical practice framework non-maleficence (before doing good, first of all ensure that you do no harm) outweighs even beneficence (to do good). This should apply equally to practitioners and patients. Iatrogenesis in whatever form is to be deprecated.

One thing amply demonstrated by the literature is that like clinical supervision reflection requires time and effort, training and resources. It is not a no cost option.

Whether you choose Schön's model which describes reflection in action (thinking on one's feet simultaneously as practice occurs) or reflection on action (retrospective analysis of an experience) or another model entirely, in truth matters little. It is the engagement in the process which is important and the model you choose must fit your needs, as reflection is essentially an analysis of one perception of an incident or perspective of an incident or happening.

However, if reflective practice is considered to be a valuable source of nursing knowledge, it must be implemented at all levels. This is a challenge to nurse clinicians, educators and their managers (Wilkinson, 1999). There is also urgent need for further research into the efficacy of differing models of reflective practice and their potential benefit to practitioners.

Reflection will not bring universal or equal benefits and there are many reflective skills which one could argue are not as prominent in the nurse's everyday bag of tools as they might be. Some (James and

Clarke, 1994) may argue that the reflectivity aspect unfairly directs responsibility for professional development directly on the individual, which is an onerous responsibility even for the most motivated. Conversely, even those most enthusiastic require skills training in self-awareness analysis etc in order to become proficient reflectors. The provision of reflective training would appear to be thin on the ground and presents a formidable challenge to the profession as a whole.

If used sensitively and with due care, reflection can be a useful and powerful tool giving insight into one's practice which is unlikely to be gleaned merely from a classroom or book. However, like all high level skills it requires training and practice in order to become proficient in the art of reflection.

Practice your reflective practice responsibly and with awareness of the ethical issues that it subsequently raises both for you and your patients.

For a further debate on the role of reflection in practice development see *The Handbook of Practice Development* (Clark, Dooher and Fowler, 2001: Chapter 4).

Case studies

The following pages contain texts provided by individuals willing to share their thoughts with the reader. They have been under no pressure to do so. However, one must remember that their reflections and any conclusions reached are essentially for each of them as individuals and not necessarily for group consumption. Assume nothing when reading their accounts, from which you may or may not learn something.

Each text has a preamble outlining the main points which can be read first or referred to later. At the end of each case study points are raised by the editors that you may wish to consider when relating the experience to your practice. Where there would be repetition (for example people illustrating the points covered earlier in the book on the nature of reflections) we have quietly edited them out. Otherwise, the accounts are as you see them.

1.

Students: seeing things with a fresh eye?

Sarah Holland

Sarah Holland Dip HE Mental Health D Grade Staff Nurse Regional Forensic Service. At the time of writing this reflective account Sarah was a third year student undertaking the Diploma HE Nursing at School of Nursing and Midwifery De Montfort University.

❖ This is a student's view of the world of practice

❖ Spending between 2–12 weeks in placement provides the opportunity to observe activity from the relative safety of a learning platform.

On commencing the Project 2000 course my two main concerns were, firstly whether I would succeed and secondly, how competent a nurse I would turn out to be. I can remember one particular Staff Nurse saying to me,

Although that wall blocking your success may seem never ending, you will soon discover that it is not impossible to climb.

These words have always stayed with me and you know what, she was right.

As to be expected it is always tough starting at the bottom. As a student nurse I felt powerless, but as new opportunities and experiences arose I found that I had the potential to offer more to the nursing profession than I had first thought.

As I became accustomed to my training I realised the importance of taking advantage of every opportunity and learning experience. Every place and area of work has its own way of doing things, if you like, its own routine, practices and procedures, each clinical area having a unique and individual feel. As my confidence grew I was able to observe and question certain practices and build up a repertoire of new skills and knowledge.

Reflecting on my first day in a clinical setting, I remember how nervous I was. It was a strange, new environment to adapt to with a new set of people to impress. I remember the unnerving feeling of whether or not I would fit in. I was both sceptical but excited and ready to do my best to make the grade. The label 'student nurse' was fixed firmly upon me and then the learning experience began.

I soon discovered that I was not this powerless, unimportant student nurse. I discovered that these learning experiences were important in that they gave me the chance to develop new skills and increase my knowledge of nursing practice.

I will be able to carry these experiences with me throughout my training, right through to becoming a staff nurse and hopefully beyond. It is these experiences that will enhance and develop nursing practice by reflecting back on good and bad experiences, adapting and improving them.

I soon realised that the more experience I gained, the more knowledge I would have to pass on to up-and-coming nurses, and the more I would have to offer to the nursing profession as a whole.

The UKCC emphasises that as a prerequisite to practice development, the practice must be sensitive, relevant and responsive to the needs of the individual patient and clients, and have the capacity to adjust where and when appropriate, to changing circumstances. For student and qualified nurses alike, practice development is synonymous with teaching and professional support, and is underpinned by research. If this is the case, it assumes that things could be better, and that the development of practice is an evolutionary process. Relating this to Benner's (1988) model all nurses could be seen as working towards expertise. As a student I am constantly acquiring and assimilating new knowledge and skills to advance my abilities in the care that I provide. This in turn will enhance my professional growth, and will be put to good use in the future.

One advantage of being a transient student nurse spending between two and twelve weeks within a placement, is the opportunity to observe the practices and interventions within a range of clinical settings. This peripheral membership of care teams limits any ability to instigate meaningful change, but provides the chance to observe activity from the safety of a learning platform.

I have noticed during my training that practice development can take place at a number of levels. In some clinical areas there was no evidence of any form of practice development. In these settings staff morale was low and the relationships between staff were poor. If staff morale is low and nurses are not supporting each other then it is inevitable that it will affect the whole functioning of the clinical area, particularly patient care.

At one particular place I visited, I noticed that the clients' daily care records, from my point of view were not very substantial, and did not reflect either the needs of those patients, or the interventions that were taking place. This was demonstrated in the record keeping which at best consisted of a couple of lines for each entry. Also staff who had hardly spent any time with a particular patient were writing in their notes. To me this is not good practice, as without evaluating care well clients' needs are not being met. This example emphasises the need to constantly monitor nursing practice and find new and more effective methods of achieving optimum care.

To me the term practice development in its simplest form means to reflect on practice, to make room for improvement. If communication between staff is good and morale is high then certain areas of care can be addressed, adjustments (where needed) could be made to aid in being more responsive to the needs of the client.

Although I am powerless to make immediate changes, as a student nurse I am building on experiences and developing practice by reflecting on these experiences. On entering the nursing profession as a qualified nurse I will be able to pass this knowledge on to my colleagues.

I have learnt a great deal from reflecting on what I have experienced during my training. It has provided me with a way of learning. I can then go on to develop these skills to become a reflective practitioner.

An example of how reflection has helped me was while on clinical placement. I was working with a client, trying to decipher any concerns and worries that this client had. I found myself getting very frustrated as he refused to communicate with me.

Throughout the day, although he still refused to communicate with me, he would come and sit with me. Each time I proceeded to tell him to go and sit elsewhere as I was busy working. This behaviour continued and after a while I decided to analyse his behaviour and discovered that by spending time with me he was building up a trust, a kind of bond with me. This was confirmed as after a period of just sitting alongside me it became evident that he had started opening up and the relationship developed from there.

On reflection I learnt that I did not fully understand the concept of interpersonal relationships, but from taking advantage of the various types of literature available I was able to make sense of what had occurred. Through reflection I was able to improve my knowledge so that if a similar situation occurred again, I could look back on this experience and deal with it more effectively for the client and myself.

To me experiences like this are good, as they are part of the learning process and it is evident that staff are often unaware of their potential in influencing or changing the context or culture in which they work.

According to Andrews (1996), in order to develop practice nurses must reflect on what they do and what they could do better. This is a prominent feature of both pre- and post-registration education programmes. As a student I especially feel that reflection is a major part of nurse training. I am constantly being reminded that it is important to integrate theory and practice, and feel that reflection has the potential to address issues in practice in a way that the straight application of theory to practice does not. Reflection can help us learn from our own mistakes as well as the mistakes of others. It can help to identify future fields for research or just make us feel better about an event or clinical incident.

At present student nurses are underrated in their ability to offer considered alternative insights to the often stale interventions administered by 'experienced' qualified staff. As novices taking our first steps in the nursing profession, our observations should be given more credibility, as it is often the naive voice which offers the freshest perspective, and new ideas are the lifeblood of practice development. I hope that eventually we will be taken more seriously and that nurses will listen to our ideas. We have more time to reflect and more time to develop the ability to reflect. The nursing profession should take advantage of this.

Key questions and discussion points

❖ Students invariably offer permanent staff an alternative perspective. What value is placed on the student's view?

❖ How can we help students learn from their clinical placements?

❖ How can we acknowledge and utilise the student contribution to the development of practice?

❖ What are the difficulties in having students with you? Students often provide a challenge which can be anxiety provoking for even experienced practitioners.

2.

A day in the life of a student nurse

Shams Uddin

Shams Uddin is now a D grade staff nurse working in acute mental health. Shams, at the time of writing, was a third year undergraduate nursing student at De Montfort University, Leicester.

> ❖ This account is an honest reflection focusing upon an elderly confused lady with multiple pathology. The discussion epitomises some everyday practical and ethical issues in health care.

Reflective practice is a complex and active process of critically examining experiences that have taken place during professional practice (Ramsden, 1997). Reflecting upon experiences with particular reference to some theoretical frameworks and research may enable health care professionals to change their own practices and interventions in positive and explicit ways (Jarvis, 1992). The aim of this chapter is to critically reflect upon a day in the life of a student nurse in an elderly psychiatric assessment ward. As a student nurse I was participating in as many different activities as I could, in order to gain maximum experience out of the particular placement allocation, as I felt such opportunities might not arise again.

The activities I participated in were wide and varied and included providing individualised care, administrative work, dispensing medications and much more. The unit could accommodate up to thirty patients at any one time. However in my opinion the staff-patient ratio was never compatible and as a result certain aspects of caring, for example, spending quality time with patients on a one to one basis, so central to the notion of individualised and holistic care, was at times overlooked.

During my allocation I was confronted with many situations that required taking a step back and critically thinking about it, while drawing upon various theoretical and philosophical understandings to rationalise what was happening. There is however one particular situation that sticks in my mind. I was involved in the care of an elderly lady diagnosed as having Parkinson's disease and dementia. She also had insulin dependent diabetes mellitus. She was originally admitted for a deteriorating confusional state and for a sudden increase in aggressive behaviour. Nevertheless, she was quite responsive, co-operative and alert at the time of admission.

A few days after admission she began to refuse both food and drink and consequently her diabetes was becoming dangerously out of control progressing to a hypoglycaemic state. She was also becoming dehydrated due to the lack of fluids. However, she appeared to me to be comfortable and free from discomfort. Both the doctors and the nurses became extremely concerned about her safety and well-being and an urgent medical intervention was felt necessary.

This intervention was the administration of 5% dextrose solution through intravenous infusion to rehydrate her. The patient was most resistive to any intervention at the beginning, however, once the treatment had started she did not struggle any further. Therefore it may be that she complied rather than consented to the treatment.

When the patient was refusing food and drink, no attempt was made to contact any family members or any other person of significance to her. Whether she was refusing food and drink because she felt rejected by her family, or that she felt lonely and frightened in a strange and busy place, or simply she did not like the taste and presentation of the meals or due to some other underlying problems was never discovered. Reduction in blood glucose was causing cerebral dysfunction (Gordon, 1982), and the dehydration was causing confusion (Malone, 1994). I believe these were significant factors that prevented this patient from interpreting what the professionals were saying, and articulating and expressing her feelings and wishes in a way easily understood by them. From a nurse-patient perspective or a student-patient perspective, I believe that contacting a family member or someone familiar to the patient would have enabled the nurses to discover if there were any underlying problems, hence this approach would have been more beneficial.

As an undergraduate student nurse whose primary role was to observe and learn, I felt powerless to make any suggestions in the presence of the professionals who were obviously more knowledgeable and experienced than I was. This placed me in a dilemma as I struggled to decide whether the actions of the professionals could be justified on the grounds that they were acting in the best interests of the patient by preventing her hypoglycaemic state from deteriorating any further or causing harm by inflicting unnecessary pain and discomfort.

Observing the look of powerlessness and a sense of failure in the hands of the professionals and the pain and discomfort caused by transferring her from one place to another in order to begin the infusion, I felt a sense of failure myself by not being able to do anything to advocate on her behalf. This caused a great deal of frustration and made me question the whole practice. This observation also inspired me to carry out a literature search and via CD ROM database I was able to obtain a plethora of literature using the keywords 'hydration, dehydration, treatment and ethics'. A comprehensive review of the literature reveals that intravenous infusion causes immense discomfort in patients, which subsequently reduces the 'good' of the act which was to bring relief.

From an ethical perspective the absolutism philosophy or 'end justifies the means' the actions could be justified on the grounds of outcome, this is her hypoglycaemic state did not deteriorate any further. This philosophy gives health care professionals firm grounds on which to stand as its main principle is; if the result is satisfactory then the methods used to achieve that result is acceptable (Edwards, 1996).

Having said that, it also raises important questions of patient's liberties and the right to make choices. However, as no family members were present at the time to advocate on her behalf, and she was not in a state to respond rationally either, then the professionals had both a legal duty and a professional obligation to act as what they perceived as being in her best interests. I believe the priority was to maintain physical stability, overlooking her emotional and comfort needs. Perhaps, there were some underlying physical, biochemical or pathological reasons behind the actions taken, although this was not explained to me. As I was left to contemplate events without any factual information I turned to research to provide me with answers.

Reflective practice is about critically examining situations that may have occurred during professional practice with a view to improving the quality and standard of care patients receive. My literature review reveals that some authors (Jones and Williams, 1993, Darbyshire 1993 and Richardson, 1995) are sceptical of this notion fearing it would become the latest fashion victim, probably because nurses are good at identifying areas of practice development but are frightened of expressing their views to those in authority. Individuals should not be frightened to express their views as this defeats the objectives of undertaking reflective practice. I realise now that I should have stated my feelings, at least it would have been worth a try.

Having critically reflected upon this situation, I make the following recommendations to enhance future care and practice.

- Upon admission a full and comprehensive assessment of the patient needs to be carried out identifying all of the details central to providing therapeutic care for that patient.

- With reference to the above patient, she should not have gone without food and drink for such a long time which under the circumstances, necessitated urgent treatment. Therefore, closer monitoring and changes in care according to circumstances needs to be implemented.

- There need to be recognised guidelines or protocols advising health care professionals of the actions to take in such situations to prevent inconsistencies in care and also to prevent patients from unnecessary exposure to pain, discomfort and suffering.

- Students and heath care workers should spend more time with patients and be an integral part in all care concerning the patients they have regular contact with. This will narrow the gap between students, support workers and qualified staff and in turn increase self-esteem and boost morale in the work place.

- All the possibilities need to be considered while having the patient in the centre of the issue before deciding upon possible actions.

- All actions need to be explained to students that may be present and health care workers for their understanding and personal and professional developments.

- Students should make an assertive effort to gain knowledge about different clinical situations they come across and attempt to analyse their interactions within the wider context of the nursing discipline.

- Reflecting upon situations using a recognised model of reflection will enable students to examine their own feelings, attitudes and knowledge about the practical, ethical and moral issues involved in nursing. This should become an integral component in every theory-practice module.

In this chapter an elderly diabetic patient became dehydrated as a result of refusing food and drink, sending her to a hypoglycaemic state. The medical intervention felt necessary was the administration of dextrose solution through intravenous infusion. From a student's perspective I believe a different approach would have spared this patient from the pain, suffering and discomfort caused by the procedure. Accordingly, a number of recommendations have been put forward for future care and practice.

Key questions and discussion points

❖ The author of this account feels that his primary role is to observe and learn. Is it appropriate for students to challenge more experienced professionals in complex situations?

❖ How do you achieve a balance between active participation and passive observation?

❖ If you were the author's clinical supervisor how would you have responded to his reflections on the difficulties experienced during this placement?

3.

Going live: The transition from student to staff nurse

Sonia Maisey EN(M) Dip HE works as a D grade staff nurse in a city general hospital intensive therapy unit.

❖ This account looks at the preceptorship period and the difficulties in transition from student to staff nurse. Although they take place in an ITC environment, the reflections are applicable to other settings.

❖ The account highlights Sonia's personal expectations and contrast these with the realities of the role.

I have recently completed a Project 2000 course Dip HE Nursing at Charles Frears School of Nursing and Midwifery, De Montfort University, Leicester. My first post as a newly qualified staff nurse is on the intensive care unit at the Leicester General Hospital. My interest to pursue this job was driven by my commitment to provide holistic quality patient care, this being one of the few areas left where qualified nurses get to deliver the 'hands on' care themselves. Following a very brief placement as a student, all of two weeks, it was long enough for me to realise that this was an area where I wanted to develop and optimise my experience within this undoubtedly challenging field of nursing. I knew that this would be a good place to build upon my practical skills as well as being able to develop the specialised skills required for intensive care nursing. During my allocation, there was noticeably a team-spirit atmosphere filled with knowledgeable, experienced staff, with many acting as good role-models. This seemed to be a perfect environment for consolidating my learning. A good place to begin, where you are surrounded by many experienced qualified staff who are motivated and enthusiastic as well as having the knowledge and specialised skills.

A summary definition of intensive care is provided by Adam and Osborne (1999).

Health care for severely ill patients with potentially reversible conditions with potential or established organ failure, commonly the lungs. The patients require close observation and/or specialised treatments that cannot be provided on a general ward. Therefore care is provided in a clearly defined area, where specialist multi-disciplinary staff and technology can be successfully combined in the management and care of these critically ill patients.

It is an area where qualified nurses make up the largest proportion of the work force. In the simplest terms the nursing role is the delivery of holistic individualised care of a supportive, preventive and therapeutic nature. Within this high technology setting, the nurse is the primary carer and the patient's advocate, which is fundamental in preserving and upholding the dignity and humanity of the patient in his or her care.

The essential qualities of the intensive care nurse are self-motivation and adaptability, not just to deal with the inherent stress of caring for the critically ill patients, but also to thrive and professionally develop within an environment which demands ever increasing standards of knowledge and practice.

At the beginning of the job my fears were about whether I would be able to master the many technical skills which were expected of me and at the back of my mind there was the fear of making a mistake.

As part of the preceptorship booklet provided were many of the clinical skills which had to be completed over a six-month period. Throughout my training I was never in an area long enough to be exposed to or master any of the skills required to nurse a patient who was critically ill or unconscious. Now I was faced with a vast range of technical equipment such as ventilators, cardiac monitoring and dialysis machines and, of course, there would be a patient as well.

No two shifts are alike, the condition of a patient can change very quickly and this can be very demanding. You can often feel like you're 'spinning plates' throughout a shift.

As a junior member of staff you are extremely dependent on the experienced staff around you and you have to rely on their patience and tolerance while you fumble your way through many of the clinical skills which they all seem to do with ease and competence.

I had four weeks of being supernumerary and I was given a preceptor to shadow. Throughout this period I continued to feel like a student, mainly observing and being supervised. There were times when I felt completely bombarded with information. I tried my best to read up at home and often before a shift began I would sit in my car for ten minutes going over my notes from the previous day. There would be days when I became so overloaded with information that I would go home completely exhausted and with a headache. My memory seemed to be affected too. I would be told something one day and forget the next.

During my training we had completed a teaching and assessing module and I had written an assignment on what can hinder learning, and I had become a text book example.

Those first few weeks of being without my preceptor, 'going live' felt like I had been catapulted into a lion's den. I was terrified, even talking was difficult. I had no confidence.

One particular day the mother and father of my patient were visiting. His sedation had just been switched off and we were anticipating his waking. I introduced myself as I had not met them before nor had I nursed their son before. After a few minutes of small talk I proceeded to continue with my necessary tasks.

His mother was chatting away to me, asking all kinds of questions. She seemed to be more interested in me than her son. His father was sat next to the mother and he had his newspaper with him. He would occasionally look up and ask the odd question or two. I was aware that I was concentrating so hard on the necessary clinical tasks that had to be performed that I knew that I was feeling more and more self-conscious and flustered and uncomfortable.

When the parents knew I had only been qualified a few months I could feel them watching me even closer. For self-preservation I had to change the subject and divert their focus away from me. So I suggested to his mother that it would be OK for her to sit closer and hold her son's hand. She could talk to him as well. I told her that although he may not be able to respond he could still hear and feel. I lowered the bed and brought her chair forward so that she was able to reach her son's hand. Her awkwardness was very obvious. She was unsure of this as I could see her hesitating. His father remained in his chair, some distance from the bed and he continued to bury his head in his newspaper. I continued chatting to his mother to help her feel more at ease. I reassured her that holding his hand and talking to him would be comforting for him.

It was at this point I began to question myself. Was I right to encourage his mother to interact like this? I had no idea of the sort of relationship they had. Some families are very tactile and like to touch, hold one another and are obviously close. That is the way I am with my own family. This family may not find it a very easy thing to do. I felt I was being too assuming. If this was my own son lying there, I know that I would be feeling helpless and if by holding his hand and talking was of some therapeutic value, then I would be prepared to overcome the feeling of inhibition that was preventing me from being able to express myself.

How did I know if I was right to encourage this behaviour? I could only assume it was the right thing to do. I had overheard other staff saying similar things to relatives, so I pacified my own doubts. On reflection I felt that I achieved what I needed to overcome my own anxiety. I was relieved that their attention was now firmly on their son rather than me, and could continue with getting on with the clinical tasks without feeling self-conscious of them watching me.

The parents appeared to be less awkward as the day progressed, and by the end of their visit his father was chatting to his son about crossword clues and his mother was giving him regular mouth care, and the atmosphere was quite relaxed between them.

However, I found the situation quite stressful and emotionally draining. My actions were out of a selfish need to preserve myself and cover my own awkwardness and lack of self-confidence to be able to perform in front of an important audience.

On reflection I learnt that I did not fully understand how best to communicate with an unconscious patient. I had become so wrapped up in myself and just getting on with the clinical tasks, I had not given sufficient attention to the psychological aspect of my patient's care, or considered the impact of the admission on his parents. The preceptorship booklet focuses on the clinical skills and very little mentioned about communication. I feel it takes a particular skill to be able to communicate with somebody who unable to respond.

This experience prompted me to read current literature about communication with unconscious patients in ICU. I also attended a teaching session on the subject.

By using reflection as a tool for learning I now feel confident that my actions were in fact justified. This has provided me with an opportunity to improve upon and develop my level of experience for future practice, even if I was acting out of instinct at the time .

Analysis of and reflection on this incident has enabled me to recognise an element of mental defence mechanisms within myself, which fortunately achieved a positive outcome. I was able to manage myself more effectively. Also I have gained confidence in a better understanding of my professional practice. The parents appeared to benefit and interact with their son in a more natural way, and from reading the current literature I learnt that communication with an unconscious patient is of great benefit as the intensive care nurse acts as a link between the patient's inner thoughts and the outside reality. With the varying levels of consciousness this aspect of care needs more emphasis.

By pursuing this I have become more aware of caring for relatives, as well as the psychological aspects of patient care, and it has led me to develop a further interest into the management of ICU psychosis and post-operative confusion.

The knowledge I have gained from this will enhance the future care I give. Being sure of what I am doing and why I am doing it provides a great sense of sincerity and satisfaction to my work.

I found the teaching session extremely informative and of great value and access to the current literature useful. I would like to see a more formal way of encouraging reflection as a means of professional development on the unit.

It would be helpful if this could take the form of clinical supervision, where individual case studies could be discussed.

When I next came on duty at handover, it was reported that sadly my patient never regained consciousness and the decision was made to withdraw treatment. Out of the eight staff on that day no one knew him or his family. I spoke up and offered to nurse him that day, but the nurse in charge felt that I was not experienced enough and it would be too traumatic for me. I was allocated an 'easier' patient that shift.

I could see his family from across the ward. I felt frustrated that I was denied the opportunity to continue with the privilege of nursing him and caring for his family at such a time, when they knew me and I had become comfortable and had built up a rapport with them. I respected the decision. The nurse in charge was primarily concerned with protecting me and I appreciated her well meaning actions.

He died later that day and I watched his family leave the unit. Unknown to them they had helped me find confidence in myself. They had been able to express their love and say goodbye to their son. It takes a particular skill to communicate with someone who is not able to respond . His mother saw me just as they were leaving I walked over to her. No words were exchanged, we just put our arms around one another.

Key questions and discussion points

- ❖ Do you remember your own first few weeks as a qualified professional? How were your experiences different from Sonia's?
- ❖ In what way has the introduction of preceptorship improved this transitional experience?
- ❖ Is there a need to 'master' the clinical skills before being able to focus on the surrounding relationship and communication skills?

4.

Nursing is not for me?

Anonymous

❖ The author of this account has been qualified (RMN, ENB 998 BSc) for ten years and has held posts up to and including ward manager level. For his own reasons he wishes to remain anonymous.

❖ Since writing this account he has left nursing altogether.

I started nursing for what I thought were all the right reasons, 'because I wanted to help people get better', 'because I thought I could make a difference'. My mother had been a nurse so I felt that through childhood dinner table anecdotes and funny stories, coupled with more serious conversations as I grew older, I knew (more or less) what I was letting myself in for.

My nursing career started with boundless enthusiasm. I was 26 when I started my training. I had already been to university and obtained a degree in engineering. I had held numerous jobs in industrial and other settings and felt that I was off to better things and was looking forward to a proper career.

My training was relatively uneventful and having already studied at degree level, I coped quite well with the academic demands of the course. After qualifying (mental health branch) I went to work on an admission ward dealing with clients from a geographical area of a large city in the Midlands.

My introduction to preceptorship, or should I say rather lack of it, occurred on my third day after taking up my staff nurses post. The deputy ward manager who should have been in charge was sick and the staffing complement for the afternoon was me (with a total qualified experience of three days), two nursing assistants and a very nervous general student (who did not want to be there) on the first week of her psychiatric secondment.

Crisis was upon me and I loved every minute of it. Never mind that the patients managed to delay tea (and visiting), that administration of the few medicines took over an hour and a patient broke a window, at the end of the day everyone was still alive. I had coped admirably and even the nursing process was filled in.

With hindsight of course, the twenty or so patients received less than adequate care from an over-confident nurse with no experience, with no one to call on should anything have gone awry.

Very soon the reality of being qualified in that environment soon dawned. Most of the staff were doing (and were expected to do) massive amounts of overtime just to maintain minimum staffing levels. In addition there were the difficult patients (in reality the least of the problems), the ward was blessed with indecisive medical staff and even less decisive managers who were not as supportive as they should have been. Some of my colleagues were too scared of the patients to be much use in teaching me what I needed to know. I felt that I should have received pearls of wisdom from the more experienced staff though they were few and far between.

By virtue of simply being there long enough and working in the acute setting, after changing wards (all acute work, as the clinical directorates system means you are stuck where you start) I found myself as a deputy ward manager after only being qualified for four years.

Now I thought I could really make a difference. Wrong again! I found myself tied up with endless juggling of the rota, staff who went sick whenever they felt like it and did not seem to care about the rest of us. I also had a ward manager whose high blood pressure and recurrent stress sickness meant that effectively after only a few months I was acting as the ward manager more often than not.

I was now in a different world, having to deal with the staff and their morale and the almost endless vacancies on one side and the 'policy directive' work delegated from the clinical nurse manager on the other. These polarised demands are difficult to reconcile; one demanded that I did more clinical work, and the other that I comment on a particular policy or sit on some working group. For the first time I started to run out of energy and my personal life suffered. I also began to feel stale. I had only attended a few internal courses since qualifying and felt the need to learn more. However, although I felt I needed more knowledge, I could not clearly identify the areas of study which would readily assist me in my daily work.

Getting on a course of any kind proved nigh on impossible and found myself in a Catch 22 situation. I could have time off if I could arrange cover (I could not arrange cover for the ward at the best of times), and my employers would only pay half of any course fee, no matter how relevant to my specialty.

After months of being overworked, understaffed and promised development I felt very disappointed. I had also failed to get a ward manager's post on a permanent basis. The reason given was partly my apparent failure to prevent a patient on leave from taking an overdose, and partly that I had not done enough post basic training. My personal life went from bad to worse, divorce was looming and my career stagnant. I began to feel bitter.

Management no longer seemed to recognise the game. It was as if I was trying to play cricket but 'they' were playing rugby. I wondered sometimes whether they recognised the nature of the beast. We deal with 'disturbed' people. Sometimes they do things that are 'disturbed'. It is not my fault.

In the absence of the ward manager who was often off sick with a variety of stress based problems, I now got blamed for anything that went wrong. Despite everything, I managed to get on a course but was constantly 'phoned to return to the ward to cover due to the shortage of staff, so it took me an extra term to complete the course and I had to fight for extra time to finish.

The clinical nurse manager left and a new manager was appointed. He was smart, cocky, arrogant and always around asking seemingly endless questions. For some reason, despite my responses to him which I think were a little curt, he seemed to like me. My ward manager retired on the grounds of ill health and I thought I might get the chance to take over. Wrong again. Suddenly I was plucked from the ward and transferred to another ward to be the acting ward manager (coincidentally the ward I first worked on after qualifying). The ward manager had just been moved to the ward I had just left. I wondered why but never found an answer to my question.

I began to be conscious that I did not possess any formal management training, but getting on to a management course proved impossible. My new ward though had a good team. With only two exceptions they all seemed to like me, I had worked there before and felt that I could really achieve something.

This is it. I have finally arrived. I can really do something now. Wrong again.

The senior medical staff dominated the scene with old-fashioned drugs and practices, petty attitudes and an inherent dislike of anyone who wanted to disturb the status quo. Rifts developed and the staff split very much down age lines, with the more traditional staff happy to stick with the old routine (less work and responsibility for the nursing staff). One or two incidents occurred, such as patients leaving the ward and taking overdoses of paracetamol that they bought while on leave.

Life at work began to be tough and I once again became disillusioned. A change round of managers meant that I had a new clinical nurse manager. In this change I lost the support given to me by the new manager, who originally I did not like but who proved to be quite supportive of his staff.

I then found myself being disciplined for the actions of my deputy ward manager when I was not even on duty. This was a crazy scenario. I protested but was told that it comes with the territory, like it, or lump it, or leave. So I was disciplined for something that happened when I wasn't even there. The excuse for this was that I should have made sure that staff were aware of procedures.

I was then turned down for yet another development course, despite the fact that there were people around me who had half the experience and been on twice as many courses. The paperwork gradually got worse and I did not seem to be able to get anything done. I felt totally unsupported though I talked to a colleague who was no help as she was even more disillusioned than I was. At this point I had been a nurse for nine years and hated the career that had promised so much and which I had started with such enthusiasm.

Eventually I could stand it no longer as whatever I did seemed to make no difference and I could see no way out of the rut. The demands of the job proved ever-increasing and the reward was more stress and no more money.

I then made a decision that I would leave nursing altogether, the politics with a large and small 'p', the paperwork and the sheer endless bureaucracy and hypocrisy of it all meant that I was finally finished as a nurse. I doubt I shall ever return to nursing and have been accepted for social work training.

Key questions and discussion points

❖ While this is only one side of the story and obviously a biased perspective, there are elements within it that sadly are all too frequently voiced by staff. Is this situation preventable?

❖ How can the health care system help people to remain committed, focused and motivated to the core issue of providing quality health care?

❖ How would you have handled the nurse if you were the person's manager?

5.

Communication is crucial in midwifery care

Kate Diamond

Kate Diamond RGN, RM, BSc (Hons), DPSN qualified as a registered general nurse in 1994 and practised for three years in the surgical and theatre setting. In 1998 Kate qualified as a registered midwife and took up a post as a staff midwife.

❖ Kate's account looks at communication, how it affects individual care and the staff who provide it.

❖ The reflection considers the difficulties of providing continuity of care in a clinically complex, multi-disciplinary setting.

Midwifery as a profession has seen many changes over the years. References to midwives were made as early as the times of the ancient Greeks. Biblical references in Genesis and Exodus describe the work done by midwives at the time.

In the nineteenth century descriptions such as Charles Dickens' portrayal of the gin swilling Sairey Gamp did little to enhance the popularity and recognition of midwives of this era. However the profession has since undergone dramatic changes.

In 1902 the Midwives Act established the Central Midwives Board which put forward guidelines to regulate the training and practice of midwives leading to their professional certification. Throughout the twentieth century as times and practices changed many amendments have been made to the original Act. However it was not until 1979 that the Nurses, Midwives and Health Visitor's Act replaced the Central Midwives Board with the United Kingdom Central Council who produce the regulations and codes which midwives follow today.

In the English language the word midwife means 'with woman'. The International Federation of Gynaecologists and Obstetricians (FIGO) and the World Health Organization's (WHO) definition of a midwife is used by the United Kingdom Central Council (1998). The midwife must be able to give the necessary supervision, care and advise to women during pregnancy, labour and the postpartum period, to conduct deliveries on her own responsibility and to care for the new-born infant. This care includes preventative measures, the detection of abnormal conditions in mother and child, the procurement of medical assistance and the execution of emergency measures in the absence of medical help. The midwife has an important task in health counselling and education, not only for the women, but also within the family and the community.

As a midwife I value this unique, professional role and the high standards of individualised care it enables me to offer. I am based in a large teaching hospital on the outskirts of the city where the client group is varied, consisting of all social groups from a variety of different cultural backgrounds. My work is based mainly in a delivery suite and a 28-bedded ward which caters for women in the antenatal and postnatal periods using team midwifery. Each day is quite varied. For instance, in one day I could spend time discussing the effects of smoking in pregnancy, caring for a woman in labour, offering help and advice with breast-feeding and give support to a family whose baby has been stillborn.

When I qualified as a midwife in 1998 I felt proud to be part of a profession which possessed the ability to understand the unique physical and psychological needs of women. I wanted the women in my care to have confidence and faith in their own bodies, and to create an environment where they could make informed decisions about their care and where I would be able to support them.

The Report of the Expert Maternity Group, *Changing Childbirth* (DoH, 1993) states that the ethos of childbirth should be that all women deserve the right to a positive birth experience and to achieve this should take an active role in decision-making, be fully informed and have care based on their individual needs. These recommendations were and still are very important in the way I offer care to women, but I have discovered that it is not always easy to practice what you believe in.

The UKCC (1992) states that the midwife must:

> *Recognise and respect the uniqueness and dignity of each client and respond to their needs irrespective of their ethnic origin, religion or personal attributes.*

Not to act in such a manner would be classed as discriminatory, yet I have discovered that discrimination does not necessarily come under the heading of sexism or racism. For example, it is often easier to give more information and choice to women who have a greater understanding and expectation of midwifery services than those who do not ask questions or take longer to understand explanations. To end this type of inequality involves more time being spent with less articulate women. However, financial and manpower constraints which lead to a lack of time and large caseloads, mean that some women are denied the care that they need.

The need for clear communication between the midwife, the woman and other health care professionals is well documented. Flint (1990) states that midwives and doctors are professionals who are 'employed to assist' the woman, and as 'employer' the woman should have ultimate say in what happens to her.

Communication is vital to the provision of both an effective and a satisfying experience for the woman and the midwife.

Tiran, 1997

As the lead professional in most cases it is the midwife's responsibility to instigate good communication. In order for a woman to experience a positive pregnancy and birth experience the midwife must fulfil the role of educator, facilitator, advocate and partner, but midwives like other health care professionals are bound by such things as their employers, policies and procedures, rules and codes of conduct, lack of time, poor staffing levels, not to mention their own personal beliefs and opinions.

The incident that I have chosen to discuss took place while I was practising within the ward area. All names have been changed in order to maintain confidentiality.

Mary was a thirty-two year old woman who was admitted to the ward during the thirty-third week of her third pregnancy, following an episode of bleeding.

Any bleeding after the 24th week of gestation and before the onset of labour is referred to as an antepartum haemorrhage or APH. There are a number of reasons why women might experience an APH. Some are extremely serious such as bleeding from the placental site, some less serious for example post-coital bleeding from an eroded cervix (erosion of the cervix can be caused by perforation of the lining of the cervical canal due to the action of hormones in pregnancy). There are several ways to diagnose the reasons for an APH. In Mary's case it was thought necessary to perform an ultrasound scan. From this scan Mary was diagnosed as having a low lying placenta or placenta previa. Placenta previa is a condition where the placenta is either partially or wholly implanted in the lower part of the uterus (lower uterine segment). The possibility of haemorrhage from a placenta previa poses a great risk to both the mother and her unborn baby, however there are varying degrees of severity. Rankin (1996) describes them as:

Type 1: The majority of the placenta is in the upper uterine segment. Vaginal delivery is possible. Blood loss is usually mild and mother and foetus remain in good condition.

Type 2: The placenta is partially located in the lower uterine segment, near to the internal cervical os. Vaginal delivery is possible however the risk of maternal haemorrhage and fetal hypoxia are increased.

Type 3: The placenta is located over the internal cervical os but not centrally. Bleeding is likely to be severe particularly when the lower segment stretches and the cervix begins to dilate in late pregnancy. Vaginal delivery is inappropriate as the placenta precedes the foetus.

Type 4: The placenta completely covers the internal cervical os and torrential haemorrhage is likely. Vaginal delivery should not be considered. Caesarean section is essential in order to save the life of the mother and the foetus.

In order to ascertain the degree of risk to the woman and her baby and plan appropriate care, an accurate ultrasound report stating the type of placenta previa is essential.

In Mary's case this did not happen. The report stated that the placenta was 'low lying' but did not state the degree of severity. Mary was scanned late in the afternoon and by the time the report had reached the ward the ultrasound department was closed. As the degree of Mary's placenta previa was unknown the registrar on duty decided not to take any risks and to treat Mary for a severe placenta previa; bed rest in hospital, where she could be observed for the remainder of her pregnancy, then delivery by caesarean section was prescribed.

Later in the evening Mary called me to her room to discuss the prognosis and the prescribed care. She was anxious about the prospect of staying in hospital until her baby was born as she had problems with child care for her two younger children. She discussed self-discharge and I explained the possible complications which could arise as a result. I suggested that it may be possible to re-scan her so that we could determine the exact position of the placenta and the degree of risk. I told her that I would discuss this with the obstetricians involved in her care.

I was due to go off duty for two days and so passed the details onto my colleges to organise.

I returned from my days off to find that Mary was still an in-patient. I discovered that my message had not been passed on and so no further action had been taken. I spoke to the obstetrician that morning, Mary was re-scanned and discovered to have only a Type 1 placenta previa and was able to be discharged home with the appropriate follow-up.

I felt that I had really let Mary down. Mary had spent the last few days needlessly worrying about her children because of a lack of adequate communication between the staff responsible for her care.

I felt angry and disappointed with the sonographer for not documenting the findings of Mary's scan accurately; with my colleagues who should have passed the message on; with the obstetric registrar for not considering a re-scan in the first place; but most of all with myself when I realised, in retrospect, that I should have made a note of the circumstances in Mary's notes for others to read and act upon.

I was pleased that Mary could be discharged home, but felt guilty that it could probably have happened sooner if my communication skills had been better. I've always considered my interpersonal skills to be of a high standard, so realising that they could improve will prompt me to examine the way that I communicate in future.

If a similar situation arose I would try to handle things differently. If the incident took place at a time when the ultrasound department was open, I would attempt to contact the sonographer involved to find out the exact findings of the scan and return the notes for an accurate documentation then contact a member of the obstetric team to discuss the correct report.

If the incident was out of hours like Mary's, I would document the individual circumstances of the woman as well as passing a verbal message via my colleagues so that any care prescribed could be done taking the woman's unique circumstances into account.

In a case of placenta previa the lead practitioner is the obstetrician. However the midwife still has a responsibility to maintain an individualised holistic approach to care by offering informed consent and acting as the patient's advocate.

Obviously I realise that nobody is perfect and that in such an unpredictable job as midwifery I won't get things right every time. There will always be constraints on the way midwives practice, but I hope that by reflecting on such incidents I will be able to improve my future practice and by doing so help create a positive experience for the women in my care.

Key questions and discussion points

❖ If Kate had been able to authorise the re-scan the patient's care would have been enhanced. Is this an area for exploration in terms of practice development?

❖ How can professionals deal with anger, disappointment and guilt in a positive manner so that it does not erode the quality of working relationships or damage one's own mental health?

❖ How do you deal with situations where your knowledge and skill exceed your ascribed power to authorise certain aspects of care?

6.
Risk management and community nursing

Dawn Holding

Dawn Holding RMN, RGN, BA (Hons), ENB Higher Award is currently employed as the team leader of a mental health community rehabilitation team (CRT).

❖ Dawn's account discusses the difficulties of managing complex situations in a community setting with long-term therapeutic relationships.

❖ It also highlights the dilemma of caring for this difficult client group and the conflict of beneficence over autonomy.

The CRT is a multi-disciplinary team comprising nurses, an occupational therapist and a clinical psychologist, with sessional input from medical staff. The purpose of the team is to provide multi-disciplinary packages of care for people with severe and enduring mental health problems in a community environment following an individual assessment of need.

The team leader's post officially comprises 75% managerial duties and 25% clinical duties which, on a day-to-day basis, is difficult to measure. An integral part of the post is the level of flexibility allowed to manage these two components to ensure that the needs of the service are met. The team leader's role includes the management and supervision of the community homeless service which consists of two outreach mental health nurses employed by the Trust and one outreach mental health nurse employed by the National Schizophrenia Fellowship.

Attempting to describe a typical day within this post is very difficult as no two days are the same. General duties may include attendance at one of the many meetings where my input is required. An example of this may be the weekly team meeting where business issues are discussed and new clients are allocated. Other meetings include; the care programme approach practice group, the monthly referral panel, the clinical effectiveness group, the community risk management group and many more. Invariably attendance at these meetings results in an accumulation of work. Alternatively, the day may be taken up with visiting clients. These may be either clients from my existing caseload, or new referrals to the service from other Directorates who require an assessment regarding their suitability for transfer to the rehabilitation services. A proportion of my time is taken up with clinical supervision sessions for both team members and myself.

Some days/weeks are exceptionally hectic and I find myself drowning under the huge paper mountain which used to be known as my desk.

Other days I find a small breathing space when I endeavour to write and/or implement any policies, procedures or standards in an attempt to keep pace with the constant change within the mental health services. At times this pace can be stressful, but challenging, with no two days being the same, and any planned activity may change in response to a crisis or client need. For me this variety and uncertainty is a positive aspect of the post which makes it interesting.

There are currently two CRTs within the Trust. The teams developed as a result of the recommendations of the Community Care Act (1990), which identified community care as preferable to in-patient care for people with long term mental health problems. At this time the community services available for this client group consisted of one community mental health nurse (CMHN), who worked with a large number of consultant psychiatrists and carried a huge caseload. As the large psychiatric institutions were contracting, people with long term mental problems were being resettled in the community. The community services had to expand in order to meet this increased demand for community care. The development of the CRTs was an integral part of the mental health services' expansion and contraction plan. I am unsure of how and why the decision was made to develop a team leader's post within the team. At the time this was, and continues to be, a unique arrangement within the Trust for community mental health teams, as the post is not discipline specific. Nurses, occupational therapists or psychologists were all eligible to apply for the post.

I have been in the post since August, 1998. Prior to this I spent seven months as acting team leader. Despite having spent five years as a CMHN within the CRT prior to being appointed as the team leader, I still had many fears with regards to my new role. I was concerned about how the other members of the team would respond to me in my new role and what their expectations would be. My predecessor had been the first CRT team leader and had developed the post and the team in her own style to an exceptional standard. She was going to be a very hard act to follow and understandably I had concerns regarding my ability to maintain these standards. In reality I had the advantage of being familiar with the team and team processes, therefore the learning curve I encountered was not too steep. However, this did not stop the process being of concern. I hoped that my appointment to the team leader's post would cause the minimum of disruption to the team while maintaining a high standard of client care. I also hoped that I would be able to carry out this new role to the best of my ability, while at the same time admitting to the people I trust when I felt out of my depth and required support. I wanted to maintain the working relationships that I had already developed within the team, but was realistic enough to realise that at times this may be difficult. In practice I have encountered some difficult situations where staff members have pushed me to assert my authority and set boundaries. At times these situations have been both difficult to deal with and frustrating, but I never believed that the job would be easy, and it continues to provide me with a challenge.

One of the many operational difficulties I encountered in my new role as team leader was attempting to introduce a formal risk management process for use within the team. The use of risk assessments and risk management processes are high on all mental health services' agendas. The Trust's care programme approach (CPA) documentation stipulates that a comprehensive risk assessment should be completed on an individual prior to their discharge from in-patient care. For many years mental health professionals have stated that risk assessments have been carried out. However, this process usually occurred in the absence of any formal documentation or procedures.

The CPA supervisory group within the Trust instructed all directorates to devise and implement a formal risk management process in a six-month period. Once devised these processes and procedures were to be presented at this supervisory group for ratification prior to implementation in the practice areas.

I joined the community risk management working group shortly after being appointed as acting team leader. This group was set up following the directive of the supervisory group to devise and implement a community risk management process. The group consisted of the team leaders from the two CRTs and a G grade CMHN from the CRT West. This group had six months to devise the community risk assessment tools, care plans and write a local policy and standard: the aim being to ensure the smooth implementation of the process, therefore resulting in an improvement in client care.

As the team leader I had to consider the timing of the introduction of the risk management process. Even though the working group had six months to devise the tools, I felt that it was important that the team as a whole had the opportunity to share their views regarding the risk assessment process and, perhaps more importantly, were aware of the impending introduction of these processes, which would hopefully result in a positive embrace of the change.

The English National Board (ENB, 1991) key characteristic number ten states that the practitioner must be able to demonstrate the ability to perform a number of skills in order to manage change effectively. These skills include understanding the process of change, acting as an effective change agent, empowering team members to participate in implementing change and incorporating a high level of reflective skills into practice. I realised the implementation of this change was not going to be easy, and I felt sure many people would be monitoring my progress to see if I succeeded and was worthy of being offered the acting team leader's post. Having had the opportunity to learn about the process of change via the use of change theories, or change strategies, I felt this was an ideal time to utilise the knowledge I had gained and use a change theory to implement the community risk assessment process. I decided to use a systematic approach and chose Karl Lewin's change theory to provide me with an appropriate tool to prevent change occurring haphazardly (1958, cited in Wright, 1989). This particular change theory has three stages, the stage of unfreezing, the stage of moving and the stage of re-freezing.

The stage of unfreezing is a cognitive one on two levels: the first level is where individuals are exposed to the idea that a change needs to occur and on the second level the system recognises that there is a problem and a need for change (Wright, 1989). As the team leader I was aware that the introduction of a risk management process was being thrust upon the team and in reality we had no choice but to embrace the change. Even though the impetus for the change appeared to be management led, there was no doubt that the lack of any formal risk management process was a problem for the team. In order to improve clinical practice the team needed to ensure that risk assessments were being completed, to tighten up on administrative procedures and, in the light of clinical governance, ensure that clinical practice is evidence-based.

During a weekly team meeting I raised the issue of the risk management processes that individuals were currently using. I asked staff for their views on the effectiveness and usefulness of such processes and to consider whether they felt any improvements could be made. I hoped that the team would realise that the current practice needed improving and would support and embrace this change while they still had an element of control, rather than waiting for the change to be imposed by the management system. On the whole the team identified that the lack of formal risk management processes was a problem requiring immediate action.

The second stage, the stage of moving, involves new responses being developed based on the collation of information. This information allows individuals to clarify and identify the problem (Wright, 1989). At a later team meeting I provided staff with written information (articles, assessment etc) about the management of risk, as well as updating staff on the progress of the in-patient risk assessment procedure. I informed staff of people within the directorate who had a particular interest or experience in the management of risk in the hope that they would attempt to ascertain the views of others. Within this second stage the proposed change is planned and initiated, so obviously this stage is lengthy. This suited us as it gave the working group time to devise the process and produce the paperwork to be used. Within this stage there are forces at work that can either facilitate or impede the process of change. These are referred to as driving or restraining forces.

The facilitating forces are known as driving forces and the impeding forces are known as restraining forces (Brodie Welch, 1979). While attempting to introduce the risk management process the driving forces we encountered included staff support for the change, support from the management system, an anticipated improvement in clinical practice and the proposed implementation alongside the in-patient services' risk assessment process. The restraining forces we observed included a lack of knowledge by the staff of the assessment of risk, a reluctance to increase the amount of paperwork currently in use and a lack of multi-disciplinary involvement. It was at this stage that the risk management package was compiled and introduced to the team for comment and amendment.

The third stage is that of re-freezing. At this stage the changes are integrated and stabilised, with individuals integrating the ideal change into their own value system which, in turn, perpetuates the idea (Wright, 1989). At this stage the community risk management process was introduced as a pilot to be evaluated in six months time. It was obviously going to be a mammoth task to complete risk assessments and care plans on all existing community clients as the team's caseload is over one hundred. Therefore, the working party felt that staff required some guidance in prioritising assessments and produced a priority list. The highest priority was given to those clients subject to Supervised Discharge (DoH, 1995), this was followed by those clients defined as high dependency under the care programme approach.

In practice, the process has been in use for approximately nine months and is constantly being evaluated. Staff views and comments are constantly being sought about the process, the questions asked and the paperwork used. As a result of this numerous amendments have been made to the process and the paperwork but there is still room for improvement. Currently the main complaint with the risk management process is the amount of paperwork involved, particularly for those clients who have more than one risk identified. The working party continues to meet on a three-monthly basis in order to constantly evaluate and amend the process, and we are currently attempting to address the issue regarding the amount of paperwork involved in the process. Throughout this process of change there were many competing priorities, the main one being the need to balance the time spent on face-to-face contact with clients and the time spent completing paperwork. In reality, client contact always wins but this often results in increased stress levels for staff when the paperwork gets out of control, as it invariably will on numerous occasions.

Having attempted to introduce this change, which appeared to be driven from the top, down, I believe the change went relatively smoothly and was embraced by most staff. The trick here was to foster ownership and adopt a bottom up approach by formulating the risk management process with the team, while ensuring it met the needs of the managers, the clients and the clinicians. Obviously all individuals had their own competing priorities, had differing organisational abilities and differing levels of motivation, therefore certain staff embraced the change more readily than others. I believe the team is still in the re-freezing stage and I do not expect the change to be fully implemented for at least another year.

As a clinician I encountered a particular difficulty with a client that caused me concern. I decided to use the reflective cycle advocated within the ENB professional portfolio (1991) to assist me to reflect upon the situation and to gain a clearer understanding. This particular situation occurred during 1998 at the client's general practitioner's (GP's) surgery.

The client I was visiting was somebody I had known for

approximately seven years (for the purpose of this exercise I shall call her Karen). I initially met Karen when she was admitted to the in-patient area where I was working at the time. I left the unit to take up a post as a CMHN and had no contact with Karen until she was discharged from the in-patient area during 1994. At this time I was allocated as Karen's community key worker. Over the years I believed that Karen and I had developed a therapeutic relationship that was built on trust and mutual respect.

During a planned routine visit to Karen's home, it became apparent that her mental health was deteriorating. Her mood was elated, she was experiencing pressure of speech and she was very irritable. Throughout the course of the visit I attempted to discuss these issues with Karen. In spite of her poor concentration she was able to describe how she was feeling extremely stressed and felt unable to manage these stressful situations. At this time we devised practical coping strategies that Karen felt would be useful to help her to manage outside of visits from her care team.

Despite using various coping strategies to manage the stressful situations encountered, Karen described feeling increasingly out of control. She gradually became more elated, irritable, suspicious and very intolerant of others. She was making verbally abusive phone calls to her landlord and the CRT team base, usually outside of office hours, where she left abusive messages on the answer machine. I received numerous phone calls from Karen's family and friends regarding her behaviour. They reported that Karen was not sleeping or eating, was cycling for many hours each day, was very irritable and generally abusive towards them when they attempted to suggest that she was unwell.

Both myself and other members of Karen's care team tried on a number of occasions to encourage her to see her doctor, to take the medication that had been prescribed and to agree to a short stay in hospital on an informal basis. Karen refused all of this as she described herself as 'buzzing' and felt that she could conquer the world.

I contacted the consultant psychiatrist and the associate worker involved in Karen's care package. The general view was that Karen needed to be admitted to hospital as her mental health had deteriorated to a level where she was perceived to be a danger to herself and a potential danger to others as a result of her unpredictability, vulnerability and explosive outbursts. As Karen was refusing to be admitted to hospital informally the only option left was to admit her to hospital under a Section of the 1983 Mental Health Act.

As her community key worker I was required to maintain a prominent role within this process. Initially it was arranged for a GP from Karen's surgery to accompany me on a routine visit to her home. When the visit took place as arranged, Karen was not at home. I left a message informing her that I had visited and arranged a time for a further visit.

The very fact that Karen had not kept her appointment with me was an indicator that her mental health had deteriorated to a level where she would avoid all psychiatric personnel, as I was generally the last person to retain contact with her.

Following this failed visit, the situation was reassessed by the care team. I was aware that Karen had an appointment with her GP at the surgery in order to obtain a sick note. It was felt by the care team that this appointment provided an opportunity to ensure that Karen had a psychiatric assessment with a view to possible treatment under a Section of the Mental Health Act (DoH, 1983).

As the community key worker it was my responsibility to co-ordinate all relevant personnel. Initially I contacted the GP who agreed to be involved in the assessment and allowed the assessment to take place at the surgery. Following this I contacted the psychiatrist and the approved social worker and arranged for their attendance at the GP's surgery at the time of Karen's appointment to undertake an urgent mental health assessment.

All of the above professionals involved in this process met at the GP's surgery ten minutes prior to Karen's appointment. This ten minutes provided time for the group to reflect upon the situation and to confirm that in this instance there was no other course of action possible. When the time of Karen's appointment came she was called into the GP's consulting room. When she walked into the room she was very shocked to see all of the mental health professionals present. She was invited to sit down while the social worker explained to her the purpose of our presence there. Initially she was uncommunicative and gave the impression of being very suspicious. As the social worker was describing reports that had been received about her recent behaviour she became very angry. She denied all of these reports and started shouting at us as a group. This was closely followed by individual personal insults, mainly aimed at the social worker. Karen was very angry towards me and kept stating she never expected this to happen.

Following this assessment Karen was placed on a Section 3 of the Mental Health Act (DoH, 1983) and all relevant paperwork was completed. The approved social worker and another member of the community team known to Karen took her to hospital for admission. In light of Karen's anger towards me I arranged to visit her the following day rather than accompany her to hospital. I made contact with Karen's family and informed them of the current situation. They expressed their relief that she was in hospital as they believed she would now be safe and would receive the treatment she needed.

This incident was important to me as I had known Karen for a long time and believed that prior to this incident we had a good therapeutic relationship. As her key worker I played a major role in instigating her admission to hospital. Having known Karen for so long I was aware of how much she disliked being in hospital as she feared that once she was in a hospital she would never get out.

I believed that Karen would hold me responsible for getting her admitted against her will and at the time I felt torn between my increasing concerns for her deteriorating mental health and safety and my awareness that I would be acting in such a way that would be against her wishes. Even though I believe I acted in Karen's best interests I was concerned about the effect this incident would have on what used to be a positive therapeutic relationship. When Karen walked into the GP's surgery I felt a mixture of guilt and relief. She was obviously upset by the incident and I felt guilty as the person who had taken the lead role in instigating the assessment. The relief I felt came from the awareness that Karen would now get the treatment she needed and that the risks she posed to herself while in the community would be minimised in a hospital environment.

When visiting Karen in hospital the following day I was a little concerned about how she would respond to me. She seemed pleased to see me but was unable to discuss the incident as she stated that her thoughts were racing and she was obviously unable to concentrate on even the most basic conversation. I was not convinced that Karen's anger had subsided, I believed she would maintain these feelings towards me until her mental health improved and she would be better able to discuss her feelings in a rational manner.

The most satisfactory aspect of this incident was the cohesive team working processes. All of the professionals involved worked towards the same goal to ensure that the situation was dealt with effectively and smoothly, while at the same time, hopefully, causing the minimum disruption possible to Karen and all concerned. Even though I felt responsible for instigating the assessment, I felt I had the support of the whole team whose professional opinion mirrored my own in this particular situation, and a consensus view was held regarding the actions to be taken.

The most unsatisfactory aspect about this incident for me was forcing Karen to do something against her will, even though it was in her own best interests. Situations like Karen's continue to remind me that as a professional who works within a mental health system, I shall on occasions be required to act as an agent of social control, even if I do not want to. Despite thinking that there is a more equal power base between staff and clients within the community, there are and will continue to be occasions where my position will require me to take control of certain aspects of the client's life. This is an aspect of my job that makes me feel uncomfortable at times but may be necessary to ensure the safety of our clients, and possibly even the safety of the general public.

On reflection I believe that this incident had a detrimental effect on my therapeutic relationship with Karen (although at the time she declined an offer to change her key worker). Once she had returned home and her mental health was stable we had the opportunity to discuss the incident at length. I explained to Karen the reasons for my actions and what the possible alternatives may have been.

I felt at this point I had to be honest and explained that if a situation arose again at any time in the future where I believed she was a danger to herself, then I would have no option other than to pursue a similar course of action. Karen stated she understood the reasons for my actions and even though she felt very angry towards me she was now aware that at the time she needed to be in hospital. Despite this, Karen used to get very nervous when I was due to visit and sat looking out of the window as she believed that I would bring another person with me to see her, or that I would send somebody else. If she ever saw a police car in the car park near her home she thought they were coming to take her to hospital. Throughout our visits we would talk about these issues and I would attempt to reassure Karen that I would be honest with her and tell her when I thought she was becoming unwell and needed to be admitted to hospital (as I did prior to this incident).

Given the opportunity, one thing I might have done differently was not to have been present at Karen's assessment at the GP's surgery. Had I not been present, our therapeutic relationship may have been preserved. This is a negative aspect of the community key worker's role that has to be carried out by somebody. Those professionals who are fortunate enough to be viewed in the role of 'therapist', rather than key worker, do not usually get involved in mental health assessments which result in detention under the Mental Health Act and so are able to maintain their therapeutic relationship.

I had the opportunity to reflect upon this incident with my manager during my clinical supervision sessions. I also used the CRT reflective practice group to share the incident with the other CMHNs in the team and to ascertain their views regarding the actions taken. I was not able to reflect on the actions taken at the time as the course of events took over and spiralled quickly until they reached the expected conclusion. I would have liked to have been able to reflect more upon what I was doing at the time. If I had, maybe the course of action would have been different, but in reality I don't think so. Despite this, clinical supervision provided me with the opportunity to discuss the incident, discuss my key working role and discuss my feelings about my actions. I felt that I had adequate support from my supervisor and colleagues who were able to provide assistance in practical areas. In reality, situations like Karen's occur on a regular basis and are expected with the nature of the difficulties the CRT clients experience. Therefore all mental health professionals face almost daily dilemmas between meeting the needs of the client from a professional's perspective and from the client's perspective. Clinical supervision provides an ideal opportunity to reflect upon these dilemmas and also obtain support and clarification from colleagues.

Key questions and discussion points

- ❖ Dawn's account makes a number of references to team co-ordination and team work. Whose responsibility is it to organise, motivate and lead a team?
- ❖ It is difficult to capture practice developments that do not have complicated technical skills attached to them. Dawn describes a role that takes practice forward, but how can we identify and develop such roles?

7.

The challenges of modern leadership: a reflective account of a day in the life of a clinical team leader

Penny Harrison

At the time of writing Penny Harrison RGN, BA (Hons), ENB 100 Cert Ed was the clinical team leader (CTL) for the Gastroenterology Process at the Leicester Royal Infirmary. This consists of two general medical wards and a gastroenterology out-patient and day care centre.

> ❖ The role of the ward sister/charge nurse, or in Penny's case, clinical team leader, is a pivotal role in professional leadership and practice development.
> ❖ This is an enormously challenging role, but we are expecting too much from one person?

My nursing background consists of experience within medicine and surgery as well as critical care. I have now held positions of responsibility within nursing teams at various trusts for the past nine years. Although I consider myself an experienced clinical nurse, hardly a day goes by without a challenge or something new that I have learnt. I find this one of the most enjoyable and satisfying parts of my work. I also believe it helps to keep me passionate about a profession that I am proud to be a part of.

I tried to think what a typical day was for me in my current role. This was much harder than I had first thought. What exactly is a typical day? Variety is the key word that comes to mind to describe a typical day in the life of the CTL. Although I believe that I work as hard as any other colleague within the nursing field, I also have great flexibility in how I manage my time and organise my working life. This is perhaps in stark contrast to many of the staff that I lead within the two wards I am responsible for.

While clinical nurses work in a flexible and responsive manner to the needs of their patients, their workload is large, demanding and does have a structure that reflects activities across the rest of the hospital. Weekdays, during working hours, can be particularly hectic as patients attend many other departments for tests and treatments. I always try to remember this when working alongside colleagues and especially if, as the clinical leader responsible for standards, I require nurses deliver high quality care, sometimes under difficult circumstances. I am always full of admiration for my colleagues who are consistently enthusiastic, hardworking and a pleasure to work alongside in such a busy environment.

Within the nursing press, criticism of how nurses do not support and care for each other is frequently voiced. Although I cannot claim to be a perfect role model of nurse/clinical leader, I do try to encourage the nursing team to have care and compassion for each other, plus extend this to other members of the team. I strongly believe that if staff are happy at work with each other, this can only make for better working relationships across the board, hopefully reflecting in better relationships with patients.

So a typical day for me might include an early start to supervise a newly qualified nurse with the drug round with her team of patients. This is followed by a brief catch-up session with the more experienced nurses (care co-ordinators) to see if there are any issues that they require assistance with. If I am not working a clinical shift with responsibilities for a team of patients, then I try to prioritise my time into 'must do now', 'must do later' and 'ought to try to do if time allows'. One of the main conflicts of demand on my time is between direct patient care within clinical practice and the responsibilities of the rest of my role. Unfortunately, just because I have my clinical practice hat on, it does not mean my other responsibilities disappear, even for a temporary period. I have frequent interruptions to my time when trying to deliver patient care. I have now enrolled the assistance of the ward clerk, who filters the calls and tries to establish whether callers need me immediately or whether calls can be returned at a later time. I frequently have lists of names and numbers with a variety of issues that require my attention once the clinical shift is completed. I try to be fair but firm over the management of my time, but unavoidably have days where I am starting 'the paperwork and phone calls' when other staff are disappearing home. A major frustration for me is not the collaboration and co-operation between different services or departments, I take this as an essential part of the role, but the managing of staff and issues that are in support services to patient care. These areas such as catering, cleaning and portering seem to throw up endless problems that I am inevitably drawn into because of the way that they affect patient care. While I recognise the large steps taken forward by such services at my Trust, the nursing staff are usually the people who have to deal with issues, because they are caring for patients (and their relatives) 24 hours a day. I have empowered the nursing teams to try to tackle issues as and when they arise, but I do find frustration with 'I'll have to sort it out with your ward manager' attitude before any action can be taken.

This assumes I am on site 24 hours per day, that the staff on the ward are incapable of resolving issues and that none of us have better things to do with our time. Examples of these issues range from the standards of cleaning on the wards to chasing stores and supplies for delivery of previously ordered items. My tip for managing this is the same as any other aspect of my role, 'immediate', 'important' and 'can wait'. I also deal more efficiently with issues after a little thought on how to resolve them in the most constructive way. I find this is less stressful. In considering the challenges of modern leadership, I have divided my role into five key areas. These are:

- clinical practice
- education
- research
- management
- other responsibilities.

For me a key challenge in developing my role, has been the concentration on clinical leadership. In *Vision for the Future* (DoH, 1993), leadership in nursing is highlighted as being a factor of central importance in the future of the profession and smooth running of the NHS. This has also involved focusing on the leading of the team of staff within the area that I work in rather than managing the team. The Oxford English Dictionary defines *'manage'* as,

> *... to have control of, to be in charge of, to manage people or business.*

This definition is based in terms that are authoritative and hierarchical. For me, modern nursing leadership is about working in a more collaborative and constructive fashion with a wide team that consists of members from different professions. The inclusion of 'leader' in the title of my role sets the scene for a modern way to lead the profession. Again, with reference to the dictionary definition, 'to lead' is defined in terms of,

> *to guide, influence, introduce, action, prepare and be a means of access to ...*

These types of behaviours are more relevant and usually obtain the desired effect more rapidly when leading the team to deliver high standards of care for patients in a busy and complex environment.

The other two words in my title, also reflect the change in role from a hierarchical way of managing a ward and the concentration of leading the team within the clinical environment. This is illustrated in the title of clinical team leader. Although nurses have worked in teams for many years, the word team within the title reflects a wider application for this principle. The *Professional Code of Conduct* (UKCC, 1992) states that we should work with the multi-professional team in a constructive and collaborative manner at all times. In my role this has also encompassed working with staff across all the professional boundaries to develop the service to meet the needs of the patients at the point of need, as and when required. For patients this means from admission to the gastroenterology centre, through the accident and emergency department, to the medical admissions unit, to the wards and to plan for a safe and effective discharge. I have now been actively involved in the recruitment, interviewing, induction and appraisal of medical staff, pharmacists, dieticians as well as the complete nursing team.

Other examples also include using the role of CTL to present issues for the nursing agenda when reviewing the service offered to patients with gastroenterology disorders at the Trust I currently work within. This was within a wide multi-professional group with representation from medicine, surgery and radiology as well as specialist support services such as stoma care and dietetics.

Clinical practice

One of the most rewarding parts of my role is actually working on the wards, assessing, organising, delivering and evaluating patient care. This is the fundamental reason that I wanted to become a nurse (since the age of six). I relish the art and science of nursing that I am able to employ in the care of patients.

While I firmly believe in practice supported by evidence (the science), I also think that the importance of 'care' cannot be under-estimated (the art) and this is frequently what our patients need and desire when they are unwell and feeling vulnerable. I aim to spend 80% of my time within the clinical area. Due to demands on my time, the frequency spent taking responsibility for a team of patients on a specific clinical shift is variable. However this time is an important way of maintaining credibility with the teams of nursing and other multi-professional staff based on the wards. It allows me to develop personal relationships with the individuals within the teams and to have a thorough knowledge about their strengths or skills that need further development. It also alerts me to any difficulties that staff may be encountering on a daily basis, facilitating a speedy resolution to issues. I can also work alongside staff to support and develop their skills in different areas of clinical practice. With the current trend to place patients into 'specialist' wards (even within general surgical and medical wards) often based on specific diseases such as respiratory or cardiovascular disorders, nurses can develop skills in a limited range of specialist areas. I believe that because of my mixed experiences, I can be used by less experienced nurses as a resource to assist them with clinical skills, to ultimately deliver higher standards of patient care.

Education

This is perhaps the part of my role that I enjoy the most. I want to teach full-time at a future point in my career, but view that education within my current role is good experience for the future. I have recently had experience in the setting up and teaching of an ENB course in gastroenterology. This has been a new, exciting and sometimes daunting experience for me. The technical register of colleges of nursing has now moved into higher education. It has been like learning a new language as well as developing new skills such as marking. At times I have definitely felt like the newcomer to the education team, but it has been very rewarding. I am fortunate in having a manager who believes in taking up such opportunities. It has been interesting having a foot in each camp. I now have a better appreciation for the conflicting demands on students of nursing as well as their lecturers.

I am particularly enthusiastic about Benner's *Novice to Expert* (1988) framework for describing learning within nursing. I subscribe to the concept of continuing to learn for an entire career. For me education is also a broad concept that fits well with nursing, a profession that is continuing to develop in scope and complexity. As CTL, education starts when new members of staff join the team. A thorough induction assists nurses of all levels of experience to start work with a new team on a strong foundation. I organise this and follow it up with preceptorship programmes, clinical supervision, development programmes and in-house training via formal study sessions and competency-based workbooks. I am passionate about the wide variety of learning opportunities that can be achieved just by working in the clinical environment.

Nurses can be encouraged to reflect on events at work, either through clinical supervision, team meetings or debriefing after critical events. With assistance to develop analytical and reflective skills, plus a tool designed to help staff to write events up, staff update personal, professional and clinical skills as part of their PREP requirements. Student nurses also require nurturing so that they can become the competent and expert practitioners of tomorrow. Within my area students are actively involved in all areas of patient care, supported by qualified nurses. This pro-active approach to students coupled with an information/objective workbook that is sent to them prior to commencing in the process, has had a huge impact on our ability to recruit newly qualified practitioners. If an atmosphere of valuing individuals within the team can be achieved and extended to students during their placements, then staff will want to return and gain experience when they complete their training/education.

Other staff who need encouragement to develop include nursing auxiliaries and clerical support staff, such as the ward clerk. These individuals form as much a key part of the team as myself or any of the registered nurses. I believe that the NVQ framework based on occupational standards impacts directly on patient care in two ways. It gives auxiliaries recognition for the quality of work that they contribute to the team. It also forms a basis for an appropriate level of knowledge for staff in a supportive role and matches this to competent practice within the clinical environment. While I recognise the importance of the national debate over use of non-registered staff within the nursing profession, I believe that the NVQ framework demonstrates one method of matching the theory/practice gap. My experience of auxiliaries who have completed the NVQ programme is that they are able to transgress this divide in an effective way. The use of competency-based training also has parallels for registered nurses. This framework can be used to develop staff in areas such as managing patients with specific disorders. Examples of this within my area include oesophageal varices and parental nutrition.

However, I am a pro-active supporter of the Project 2000 styled training for nurses, as I believe that newly qualified practitioners have many skills that will assist them in their future career. These staff have very particular needs. I do feel that they lack clinical expertise and experience and have to learn these elements of practice very rapidly once they are working within the clinical environment.

The first six months of practice is a crucial time for them and I believe the one that modern leaders such as myself can impact on most effectively. I try to encourage these nurses that their education has now really begun and that they have a wealth of opportunity to take this as far as they feel they want to. I do make it clear that they also now have responsibility for their own professional development, even if they require my assistance with accessing relevant information or planning their study time.

Research

My own level of awareness and ability to use analytical skills to interpret research findings has had to be developed over the years. I have also had to combine these skills with the behaviours outlined in the management section to facilitate using the research findings and translate them into current practice. This has sometimes challenged the *status quo* or ritualistic practice. The clinical examples of this are many, from assisting patients with mouth care to humidification of oxygen therapy. However, I am glad for my background of experience because it has helped me to understand how other staff can find research a difficult concept to apply to their clinical environment. I am able to encourage them with their own anxieties or questions about applying research to practice. This is not to suggest that I am an expert at research, but I do consider myself well-skilled at acting as a role model or facilitator to the team on the ward.

Under this heading I also include evidence-based reviews and audit. I believe that these are two good tools for assisting nurses to look at current practice and review the benefits of care that we give. You can also use these aspects of work as examples of skills that can be developed and reflected on for nurses to use to meet their PREP requirements. I use an introduction to audit session, by asking staff to audit how well they have wrapped up a secret present for another individual. When the laughter has died down, nurses are surprised at how easy principles of audit can then be transferred to looking at clinical issues. As a CTL, I have successfully used this technique to review how effective the nursing team is at using admission documentation and care plans. Findings are then owned by the team and action can be agreed upon to meet areas of need. For the team I currently work in this included complete revision of the care plans we used and development of core care plans.

Management

In considering the part of my role that encompasses management, I feel it is helpful to consider where nursing as a profession has come from in recent times in terms of the way that it is managed. My current role of clinical team leader was developed from the best part of the traditional sister's role, plus a review of what is actually appropriate for a nurse to manage within a ward environment. In the mid-eighties onwards, sisters became ward managers, and embraced management roles such as having 24-hour continuing responsibility for wards, plus financial responsibility for the ward budget, which had been previously been the nursing officer and nurse managers areas of responsibilities. Within the Trust where I currently work, process management has tried to address this issue. The process manager has financial and continuing responsibility for the ward area. My contribution is to ensure that I lead the team in managing resources effectively. For example, utilising staff to the optimum level to meet the needs of the service, or ensuring that the nursing staff use the correct assessment criteria before hiring a specialist pressure-relieving mattress to prevent unnecessary expenditure.

While I recognise the importance of financial and resource management, it is helpful to have a manager who manages these aspects of work. This means that my expertise remains in the field that I was originally trained for, nursing. I feel that my current role uses many management skills in running an effective ward, but also allows me to do what I actually came into nursing for, to care for patients. After all, I trained as nurse, not an accountant or personnel manager. For me the skills required to manage the area I am currently responsible for are varied, but include:

- leadership
- negotiation
- personal
- professional
- process
- team working
- planning and organisation
- facilitation
- change management.

As well as these skills, behaviour also plays an important part in being a successful leader, including:

- enthusiasm
- persistence
- being approachable
- humour
- caring for colleagues
- communicating
- stamina
- personal development
- acknowledging mistakes.

Other responsibilities

I wondered what comments I could make about this. However it strikes me that many nurses have encounters at work that probably have little or nothing to do with nursing. As we are the professionals who have contact with the patient for 24 hours a day, it seems that nursing staff are often asked to assist in resolving unusual situations. The most striking of these that I recall is the time when two elderly patients were admitted to the ward following smoke inhalation after a house fire. In addition to the two new human admissions was a canine admission. The elderly couple's pet dog (much loved, but equally as elderly and coughing almost as much as its human companions) was also admitted to the ward. As the directorate bleepholder, I felt I had the skills and experience to sort out this challenging situation. Four hours later I finally managed to arrange temporary accommodation for the four-legged patient and a twin-bedded side room for the two-legged patients. In the time I had spent organising these unusual admissions much laughter and effort had gone into the canine assessment, care plan and drug chart. Just how do you give a dog a nebuliser, if necessary?

What would the UKCC have to say about this particular aspect of SCOPE of practice? (One of the best aspects of nursing is the silly banter and humour that comes as working as part of a team, often in very stressful situations.)

As you can imagine, resolving this particular situation had nothing to do with nursing in its purest sense and yet capsulated everything that is nursing. It was perhaps a good example of meeting patients' physical as well as psychological needs. If you had lost all your worldly possessions and nearly your life, then a pet dog becomes very precious indeed. On reflection, I felt very humbled by this experience.

So what is the future for nursing? I do think that there will be some key areas of challenges for nursing as a profession in the new millennium. I think these will include:

+ continuing difficulties with recruitment and retention of nurses, especially qualified staff with experience
+ increasing workloads and activity
+ increasing expectations from the public over standards of care

- increasing expectations from nurses that they will contribute further to patient care in partnership with the whole multi-professional team, rather than continuing to be dominated by doctors
- further moves towards a graduate-based profession.

What nurse's contribution to these areas will be, can only be imagined. I hope that I am there for the profession with a voice that represents the important issues for staff who deliver care at the sharp end.

Key questions and discussion points

- ❖ Has the nursing profession taken the distinction between management and leadership seriously?
- ❖ How do you think this role that Penny describes could be developed into that of a nurse consultant?

8.

Complementary therapies and independent practice

Gordon Gadsby

Gordon Gadsby PhD, BA(Hons) RGN, RMN, Dip.N (Lond), MISBM, DHP, DHS is a nurse practitioner/lecturer in complementary therapies.

❖ This is a reflective account of the transitional process from hospital nursing to complementary therapy practice. It describes a fundamental change to the practice of acupuncture within the framework of the therapeutic relationship.

This reflective account describes the transition process from NHS hospital nursing, as a clinical night nursing officer, to a nurse practitioner of complementary therapies within a private care practice. After twenty-eight years of hospital practice and following a period of training in biophysical medicine, which centred around acupuncture and electro-acupuncture, I decided to leave the security of the National Health Service in 1985 in order to set up my own private practice. Over the past fifteen years there have been many developments and changes to both clinical and managerial practice in complementary therapy, and this account examines some of the most important changes which have been made within my particular scope of practice. This reflective account may also help others who are contemplating such a change for themselves, or for nurses who are interested in implementing one or more complementary therapies within their own area of clinical expertise.

- **Acupuncture** is an ancient Chinese system of healing. It is based on the theory that energy flows through the body via meridians or energy channels. Pain and disease occur when there is a blockage or imbalance within this meridian system. Acupuncture points, which lie along these meridians, are treated using needles to restore this imbalance.

- **Electro-acupuncture** is a modern technique whereby electrical stimulation is applied to the needles in order to promote a return to normal energy balance. This is seen as a more effective and modern method of acupuncture treatment.

- **Hypnotherapy** is the conscious use of the natural trance-like state of hypnosis. Using the power of direct or indirect suggestion, it is a method for influencing the unconscious mind, in the treatment of physical and psychological illness.
- **Reiki** is the Japanese art of healing by the laying on of hands. A Reiki Master attunes Reiki healers to the higher healing energy source at three levels of practice.

As a nurse practitioner of complementary therapies my work entails the use of electro-acupuncture, in its various forms, together with hypnotherapy and Reiki healing where indicated. I work within a therapeutic relationship framework in order to address the physical, psychological, social and spiritual dimensions of patients seeking my help. The wide range of disorders I treat are similar to those of most complementary therapy practitioners (Vincent and Furnham, 1997), ie. patients with musculo-skeletal disorders, sports injuries, neurological pain, a wide range of stress-related problems, anxiety, depression, addictions, women's health and men's health and chronic fatigue syndromes.

On an average day I would see around six patients either seeking help for the first time or attending an ongoing course of treatment. I specialise in the treatment of musculo-skeletal and neurological pain and half my patients suffer from either acute or chronic back pain. Each patient is allocated a one-hour treatment session and first time patients are allocated up to one and a quarter hours. New patients are allocated more time so that they can tell their story, undergo biophysical tests, pain assessments, range of movement assessments, and for me to make a complementary diagnosis, construct a treatment plan and carry out the first treatment. The remainder of the working day includes clinical, academic and management administration together with ongoing research projects and forward planning.

This work developed from my long-standing interest in acupuncture, following US President Nixon's well publicised visit to China in the early 1970s, and the subsequent developments in alternative medicine in general that followed. Following my own training in biophysical medicine and electro-acupuncture in the early 1980s, and with the development of a part-time clinical practice, it was inevitable that I would eventually consider expanding this work to a full-time basis. The decision to expand my practice to full-time and terminate my employment within the NHS was made in 1985 at a time when yet another NHS reorganisation was imminent. In order to pre-empt the stress of yet another round of reorganisation I made this decision in the hope and anticipation that I would be able to survive the initial months of practice, with enough patients seeking me out for treatment to make it a viable proposition. There were of course the usual anxieties and fears to consider, such as I might not succeed and how would I manage to cope with a young family to support, a large mortgage to pay, and would this be the end of my nursing career and so on. However, these fears were quickly overcome as I found a steady supply of patients looking for treatment, either in the clinic or for home visits and I have never looked back. While there have also been some quiet times over the years, with effective time management, this has allowed me time to study on a part-time basis for my first honours degree in health studies. Subsequently over a period of six years, an MPhil and PhD followed in electro-analgesia: historical and contemporary developments.

There were very few initial strategic or operational difficulties on transition from hospital nursing to private complementary therapy nursing. The clinic set-up, client base and accounting had already been established over the preceding five years of part-time practice. However, in order to increase my client-base I decided to advertise my services in the local newspapers, magazines, yellow pages etc. This was not a successful or cost-effective venture for attracting suitable patients interested in complementary therapies and was discontinued after a few months. This initial advertising seemed to attract a few unsuitable patients, eg. people with social problems, long-term mental health problems, drug addicts and alcoholics etc. This group of potential patients was not entirely suitable for this approach to treatment, especially within a home-based clinical situation, and was also not in a position to pay for it. On reflection, the best form of advertising can now be seen to be based on a range of successful treatments and satisfied patients who went on to recommend others for this treatment.

In the initial setting up period of the practice it seemed appropriate to inform other health professionals, eg. by mail-shots to GPs, hospital consultants etc., and the general public, eg. by giving talks to interested groups of the services I was offering. However, this cannot be seen in retrospect either as a reliable or dependable procedure for attracting new patients. Other practical issues related to maintaining effective patient records and their security. This entailed increasing the clinic security with added door locks and alarms and developing simple but comprehensive accounting records. It was also necessary at this stage to find a comprehensive surgery and professional indemnity insurance. A distinct advantage of becoming self-employed was of course the comparative ease in claiming tax-deductible expenses in comparison with employment within an organisation. A further advantage of working from home was the extra time available for work and study. When there is no daily commuting to do, this extra time becomes extremely useful, especially so once I had decided to follow a more academic approach to my work and life. Once the above organisational issues were addressed I could concentrate on patient treatment. Over the years the numbers of patients increased at a steady rate to the level where I could make a satisfactory living and follow my academic pursuits at the same time.

There were few people-based difficulties within this structure, probably because I was working as a lone practitioner. There was, however, at this time a distinct lack of professional support from the biophysical medicine-training organisation both during the training course and on course completion. This organisation, now defunct, appeared more concerned in making money than supporting its members. Nevertheless, several nurse members once trained got together and formed an unofficial peer support group to give each other mutual encouragement and to facilitate discussion. This was a most helpful development to many of us, even if it had no official standing. This aspect of professional guidance and supervision, with the formation of a new training facility, has now been considerably improved and support and advice is freely available to students and trained practitioners alike from the author of this review.

In order to improve my academic knowledge, clinical expertise and professional development I also attended several post-graduate courses at this time on advanced electro-acupuncture — diagnostic and treatment techniques. I felt at this stage some difficulties when dealing with psychological problems, and in order to improve this aspect of practice I enrolled for a course of training in hypnosis and hypnotherapy and psychology and psychotherapy. It is only recently, however, and with the increased interest in holistic practice and the spiritual aspects of healing, that I followed a course in reiki healing to Reiki Master level. These three therapeutic techniques have now enabled me to provide a more holistic approach to practice taking into account physical, psychological and spiritual aspects in greater depth and within the therapeutic relationship. Ongoing professional and academic development continued throughout the following years with a BA(Hons) degree in health studies and a PhD in electro-analgesia as described earlier.

I was already aware of the importance of the therapeutic relationship within the nursing encounter, developing rapport, providing care, warmth, positive regard and support etc. However, I was not immediately aware of how important this relationship was going to be within the framework of complementary therapy practice. This knowledge was to come much later. I realised, at an early stage of practice that the ethos of complementary therapies centred on promoting self-healing and self-help. It soon became apparent that a large proportion of patients was not only looking for effective treatments but also looking for time to discuss their problems on a psychological, social and spiritual level. To this end I began to allow extra time for this aspect of care, so that patients could tell their story, discuss, accept and interpret individual views of illness and those of other health care practitioners involved in their care. I have always believed that nurses, through their training in whichever speciality, gradually develop the ability to create very effective therapeutic relationships. This includes promoting realistic hope, reassurance, acceptance, encouragement, understanding, to be good listeners, to explain and give reliable information to patients and so on.

However, I was not really consciously aware of the high degree of importance of this therapeutic relationship on physical, emotional, and spiritual dimensions until I started writing this reflective account in detail. This aspect of care was also further reinforced and extended by reading the book *The Therapeutic Relationship in Complementary Care* (Mitchell and Cormack, 1998) which encapsulates the dynamics of the therapeutic relationship so well. I was aware to a lesser degree, through my other research interests, of the power of other non-specific effects central to healing. These included the dynamics of the patient/practitioner interaction in respect of the placebo effect, the role of practitioner status, the credibility and power of the treatment ritual, spontaneous remission of symptoms and so on, but it had figured less in my conscious clinical thinking up to the present time.

While most of these aspects of the therapeutic relationship remained hidden from my conscious thinking, during the time under consideration and for some considerable time thereafter, almost all my patients were responding positively to the biophysical medicine approaches of diagnosis and electro-acupuncture treatments with supportive psychotherapy as needed.

So everything seemed to be going very well at this stage, patients were responding to treatment, new patients were seeking treatment but why did I feel the necessity to reconsider my approach to treatment. Underlying this success and as I became more skilled and confident in practice I also became aware of a surprising number of patients who would have preferred not to be needled at all, if there had been an alternative method of administering the treatment. So should I ignore these observations and my own feelings of uncertainty, for everything was going well and why should I rock the boat or should I now think seriously about investigating alternative aspects of treatment?

The above observations lead me conveniently on to a reflective focus on patients and practice. I have chosen the issue of needling patients that I felt at the time needed to be examined and resolved, ie. whether to use needles or surface electrodes for effective electro-acupuncture treatment. I was already aware of the feelings of some of my patients and also of some of the potential problems of needling as indicated below. I felt increasingly uncomfortable with the concept of the current invasive procedures if a more simple and less invasive approach could be shown to be as effective and perhaps even more so. I struggled with these thoughts for a while. I found it difficult to consider abandoning a therapy, which had cost me a considerable amount of time, effort, and not least several thousands of pounds of hard-earned nursing money to learn. At the same time I was experiencing some conflict surrounding the traditional Chinese medical theories of illness, relating to energy imbalances and blockages, meridian theory and acupuncture points. These concepts were all at variance with western science and my own nurse training. Moreover, I felt the need to consider those people who were not really suitable for needling. These included patients with diabetes, bleeding disorders or on anticoagulant therapy, HIV or hepatitis positive, people with a needle phobia, young children, or those who would just prefer a less invasive technique.

This issue gradually became more important with the increasing publicity of the late 1980s surrounding HIV and hepatitis infection and their possible transmission through needles. There was also the risk to practitioners like myself to consider from needle-stick injuries and possible transmission of blood-borne pathogens.

Before I examine the issues surrounding this aspect of practice it is perhaps a convenient time to consider some of the quality issues relevant to that time. While, again, I was not consciously aware of the dimensions of quality performance, on reflection some of them can now be identified as follows.

Firstly, was I doing the right things in my practice in respect of efficacy and appropriateness?

- **Efficacy** being the degree to which the electro-acupuncture interventions had been shown to accomplish the intended outcomes. There was no doubt that patients who had not responded to conventional approaches for pain and stress-related conditions were getting better with electro-acupuncture treatment.
- **Appropriateness** being the degree to which the treatment was relevant to the client needs. In the early 1980s patients were beginning to seek alternative and effective treatments for conditions which had not responded to conventional approaches. Acupuncture and electro-acupuncture suddenly became of interest to patients and the only problem here seemed to be the one relating to needling versus non-needling techniques, and this is discussed below in some detail.

Secondly, was I doing the right things well in respect of availability, timeliness, effectiveness, continuity, safety, efficiency, and respect and caring?

- **Availability** being the degree to which appropriate interventions are available to meet client needs. Electro-acupuncture interventions were seen as appropriate for treating pain and other physical conditions not responding to conventional approaches, but perhaps not completely appropriate to giving complete holistic care to body, mind and spirit.
- **Timeliness** being the degree to which the intervention is provided at the most beneficial time to the client. Transferring from part-time practice to full-time practice which now also included evening appointments thereby providing treatment opportunities at times that were most beneficial/convenient to my patients.
- **Effectiveness** being the degree to which the intervention is provided in the correct manner to achieve the intended client outcome. The established technique of electro-acupuncture was initially provided in the conventional manner using needles to achieve the intended outcomes of illness improvement, pain relief and stress management.
- **Continuity** being the degree to which the interventions are co-ordinated between organisations, among care providers, and across time. This was a quality issue not directly considered in view of the organisation of private practice and the lack of co-ordination between other care providers at the time.

- **Safety** being the degree to which the risk of an intervention and risk in the environment is reduced for both client and health care provider. This is one of the quality issues under consideration in this account as I examine the change from needling techniques to a less invasive and risk-free intervention strategy, for both patients and practitioners, by using surface electrodes rather than needles.

- **Efficiency** being the degree to which care has the desired effect with a minimum of effort, expense or waste. The use of electro-acupuncture has been shown through randomised controlled trials to be twice as effective as traditional acupuncture needling techniques. Electro-acupuncture through surface electrodes (now known as Neuro-Electric Acupuncture or NEAP in China and the USA) was now shown to be just as effective as electro-acupuncture through needles. Therefore, this new approach to acupuncture is more therapeutically effective and cost-effective for patients and reduces the average number of treatments required by fifty per cent.

- **Respect** and caring being the degree to which clients are involved in health care decisions and are treated with sensitivity and respect for their individual needs, expectations and differences by health care providers. One of the strengths of both complementary therapies and private practice is the quality time available for patients and practitioners to examine with some sensitivity their physical, psychological and spiritual dimensions of the presenting problem. Empowerment of patients in the treatment, decision-making process and outcome evaluation is also part of this experience.

This review of the quality issues of the time leads us conveniently on to the next stage of this reflective account and the development from this initial stage of electro-acupuncture practice to a less invasive approach to treatment.

The electro-analgesia literature of the early 1980s suggested that there was no significant difference in the degree or duration of analgesia achieved between classical electro-acupuncture and low frequency transcutaneous electric nerve stimulation (Abram, 1983). Later studies also confirmed these findings (Cheng, 1987). The clinical experience of needle electro-acupuncture and the potential problems of using needling methods, eg. bleeding, bruising, pain, pneumothorax, infection etc. led me in the intervening years to consider implementing a less invasive method of electro-stimulation. This approach would entail surface electrode placement to acupuncture points in order to replace needle insertion. At the beginning of 1990, I again reconsidered this approach in more detail and decided to plan its implementation and integration into my daily practice.

But how would my patients both old and new accept this change in procedure, and would I be thrown into even greater conflict with my acupuncture training? After some considerable thought, consideration and planning I decided to introduce this less invasive needle-less technique of electro-acupuncture to my patients on a trial basis. After all, the literature available from controlled and uncontrolled trials appeared to support this approach to electro-acupuncture, in the form of acupuncture-like TENS treatment.

This was a conclusion drawn perhaps from a less than exhausting literature search of the day. Today of course the foundations of evidence-based health care practice are more solidly laid down, through for example the work of the Cochrane Collaboration, and would now enable a more systematic review and meta-analysis of the literature to be carried out.

In the first instance I decided to introduce the needle-less procedure to some of my existing patients and then to assess their response to treatment and their thoughts about the new procedure. To my surprise this group of patients was most supportive and even expressed their approval of preference to the needling methods. This encouraged me to rapidly introduce this technique to all my new patients as they came into the clinic. They had already been informed when booking their appointment that this was the treatment protocol in use at this clinic. This approach seemed most acceptable and no patients cancelled their appointments. In fact, several expressed some relief that needles were no longer used. Within a few weeks I had abandoned the use of needles altogether, as the treatment outcomes were comparable, if not superior, to traditional methods, ie. fewer treatments seemed to be needed per course. This is the approach to treatment I have maintained to the present day. I have to admit that at the time I felt most apprehensive about making such a controversial change to practice and abandoning a technique based on 3000 years or more of observational evidence. The therapeutic results of this change in clinical practice had not reduced the beneficial effects of electro-stimulation of acupuncture points. It had in fact enhanced it and this led me then to debate within myself the basic assumptions surrounding traditional acupuncture. The ancients had painstakingly observed their patient's response to treatment and had laid down theories of health based on energy imbalances within a metaphysical meridian system. They had considered the relationship of man to the cosmos and the elements and described a complex treatment interface of acupuncture points to balance these energy imbalances. However, in the face of twentieth century knowledge might these interpretations be incorrect? While we cannot fail to admire the powers of observation of these early physicians, can we really accept these metaphysical theories without challenge when even the Chinese Academy of Science has recently proclaimed itself in opposition to superstition and pseudo-science (Shen, 1997).

Around this time the endorphin response theory to electro-stimulation were gaining ground among western and eastern scientists. This possible mechanism of explanation for the effectiveness of acupuncture was put forward, and this scientific evidence seemed to fit in more with my view of the world. This was in preference to the metaphysical Chinese meridian model of health and in spite of my reluctance to let go of it as identified above. Researchers both in China and in the West have subsequently strengthened this approach. Numerous studies have now confirmed and determined that the gene expression of endorphins and other neurotransmitters was electro-frequency specific. To this end my practice became increasingly based on the neuro-endorphin responses with their analgesic, anti-inflammatory, immune strengthening, fatigue lifting and stress reducing properties.

While this initial research knowledge was somewhat sparse and difficult to identify in the early 1990s, subsequent research publications have since verified that this approach was absolutely correct both from western and Chinese perspectives (Ulett, 1998a). This most recent review, based on more than thirty years of research in China and the West, confirms the approaches I have described above as being absolutely correct. It goes on to explain the rationale of electro-stimulation of acupuncture points, even though this knowledge was incomplete and unavailable to me at the time of implementation of these approaches within my own practice. So these innovative approaches to treatment have stood the test of time over the last decade and have now been validated by recent eastern and western research as absolutely correct.

This reflective account has examined both traditional and contemporary theories of acupuncture in relation to changing clinical practice to benefit both patients and practitioners. We can learn from this analysis that new evidence should lead us to challenge long-held beliefs and assumptions in order to enhance our future practice. In the final analysis all knowledge is provisional and we need to act on new evidence as it arises in order to benefit our patients. This new and revised approach to electro-acupuncture, by integrating new knowledge with previous knowledge, has for many practitioners, both in the East and the West, changed their practice forever. In my judgement there can be no going back to a more primitive method of treatment. The evidence from high quality research, theory and clinical practice demonstrates the superiority of this new approach to health and healing within the framework of acupuncture practice and the therapeutic relationship. It is also most interesting that as we have entered the new millennium the more orthodox of British acupuncturists are now seeking information on this new approach from practitioners like myself. Will they too abandon the use of needles and forsake the Chinese metaphysical theories of the past? Only time will tell but it does seem inevitable that this trend will continue both in the East and in the West both for today, tomorrow and far beyond. Moreover, this approach is now being vigorously promoted in the United States of America, under the new style of neuro-electric acupuncture. Its exponents are lobbying the medical schools to include this training in the undergraduate curriculum (Ulett, 1998b). Will we see this happening in the more conservative medical and nursing schools of the United Kingdom? Again, only time will tell us.

In conclusion, this reflective account examines my approach to the change from hospital clinical nursing to complementary therapy nursing. It examines the abandonment of metaphysical knowledge for a more acceptable scientific basis to acupuncture practice, as it has developed over the last few years. Perhaps these changes initially were a matter of trial and error to some degree and there was no one readily available to ask for professional help, advice and support at the time. It would have been useful to be part of a support group of like-minded nurse practitioners, such as the RCN complementary therapies interest groups and the many local NHS Trust complementary therapy interest groups of today.

I would have liked and appreciated the benefits of further discussions with a much larger, interested and dedicated nursing peer groups some years ago. However, it should be easier now for nurses who wish to pursue these approaches within the framework of current nursing interest and with the subsequent implementation and integration into practice of appropriate nurse-led complementary therapies. This is a rapidly growing and developing trend, which will hopefully continue well into the future but we now have to consider the nursing options before us. Do we provide an extended holistically-based nursing care service, which includes the use of complementary therapies within the framework of the therapeutic relationship? Or do we continue the current trend towards a more medically orientated model of nursing care, as we take over those aspects of medical practice that junior doctors no longer wish to do or have time to carry out within their allotted hours of work (Cole, 1998)? The choice is ours but which path will we choose to take – the future will reveal all.

Key questions and discussion points

❖ Gordon's move from nursing in the NHS to an independent complementary therapist was at least partially motivated by NHS reorganisations and restrictions on nurses to practise independently. Do we have the same culture today as Gordon experienced in the 1980s?

❖ In an environment where health care resources are finite where do complementary therapies fit in today's NHS?

❖ Do we provide an extended holistically based nursing care service, which includes the use of complementary therapies within the framework of the therapeutic relationship?

9.

Implementing a screening programme for fifteen-year-olds

June Freehan

June Freehan RGN, RHV, RM, BA (Hons), ENB Higher Award is a health visitor with a number of years' experience and has worked in a variety of health visiting settings.

❖ This account describes the setting up of a health screening clinic for fifteen-year-olds, reflecting on its functions and effectiveness during the first year.

Health visiting has undergone many changes since I qualified over 17 years ago. Having worked briefly as a midwife, in my new role I envisaged the opportunity to develop my existing skills and provide ongoing continuity of care to mothers and their families. It was generally understood that health visiting focused mainly on the under fives, although our remit was 'from the cradle to the grave', underpinned with specialised training to promote health and well being among all age groups within the general population.

During my early health visiting days, routine home visiting of young children was considered an appropriate way to assess child development, observe for signs of child abuse or neglect, and facilitate interventions where necessary. Frequently, health visitors developed very close relationships with the parents of children on their caseloads, while visiting them at six-monthly intervals or as required, depending on the family's needs. Community clinics also provided a social and supportive environment for young mums, where they could have their babies weighed, obtain formula milk and discuss a variety of issues with a health visitor.

In recent years, home visiting has been considerably reduced and the under fives are assessed at key stages in their development as part of the child health surveillance programme. Health promotion and assessment of children follows the recommendations of David Hall, who chaired the joint working parties on child health surveillance (Hall, 1989; Hall, 1991; Hall, 1996). In addition, the introduction of the Parent Held Child Health Record has been influential in establishing a working partnership with parents. Much of the assessment process now occurs in surgeries, under the jurisdiction of general practitioners. Child health clinics are organised on the same premises, where families are seen by their named health visitor. One of the most enjoyable aspects of health visiting is the variety of the work involved. It would be impossible to describe a typical day, since much of our work is in response to the needs of families whose child/children are on our caseloads. A telephone call from a concerned parent may prompt a visit to discuss how to manage a distressing behaviour problem, or help a mum who is having difficulties feeding her new baby. In practice, most health visitors need to plan their work carefully, in order to fulfil clinic commitments, including child health surveillance, immunisations, and many undertake group work with post-natal and ante-natal mothers, or organise sleep management clinics and weaning groups. In addition to the above, many of the contacts with clients will be centred around minor ailment and safety advice, nutritional information, toilet training and parenting skills. Other work includes; giving extra support to families who have a child with special needs, child protection involving frequent contact with a 'child at risk', attendance at case-conferences and liaison with other professionals. As part of our role in primary prevention of ill-health, health visitors are often involved in a variety of community and national initiatives promoting health and well-being. This includes presentations to different groups where, for example, we discuss ways to stop smoking, to reduce stress, to keep active and healthy and breast awareness.

The implementation of the Government White Paper, *Working for Patients* (DoH, 1989), and GP fund holding, has had a significant impact on all community nurses. Health visitors have needed to develop closer working relationships with GPs, and liaise with the practice regarding referrals to other agencies. Additionally, health visitors have had to adapt and develop their roles to meet the needs of the practice. New clinics have been established within surgeries, and we have had to find creative ways of working alongside our medical colleagues, while meeting our clients' needs at the same time.

In many practices, health professionals have been trying to address some of the health targets identified in *The Health of the Nation* (DoH, 1992), including heart disease, cancer, mental illness, HIV/AIDS and sexual health, and accident prevention. From a health visiting perspective, this and other health policies, provide exciting opportunities to develop health promotion skills with different groups of the population.

However, while the majority of health visitors are capable of tackling these issues, there is no extra funding or resources available. There is an expectation that child health surveillance will be carried out, families of children with complex needs will be supported, and parents will continue to make contact regarding issues of concern to them. These may relate to social and financial problems, relationship difficulties, and many will need additional support at particularly stressful periods in their lives.

Organising clinics and appointments is time-consuming, and there is usually a mountain of paperwork to address. A new child protection incident may also trigger hours of intense involvement with a particular family. Long telephone conversations with social services and other agencies may take place, and attendance at case conferences and core group meetings is mandatory. Sometimes finding the time or energy to think about taking on additional responsibilities is incomprehensible.

In some instances, it is relatively straightforward to respond to a community health initiative. Occasionally we are approached by an organisation or local group to give a presentation on a health issue, or to take part in a health fair. In this instance I would simply note the date in my diary and fit any preparation for the event around my other commitments. It is another matter entirely to consider embarking on a new initiative. The project needs to be thoroughly researched and planned, and the idea 'sold' to colleagues and managers. Additionally, ways of evaluating the activity and measuring outcomes need to be considered. Enthusiasm and foresight are fundamental assets.

A number of my colleagues have risen to the challenge of tackling different health needs in their practices and in the community. They have focused on a variety of issues including cardiac rehabilitation, stress management, asthma, behaviour modification and menopause clinics. Personally, I have developed an interest in the health of young people. During a professional meeting a health visitor discussed her attendance at a conference where adolescent health was highlighted as an area of concern. Until recently, the particular needs of young people were not being addressed — most were treated alongside children or adults. It is now recognised that teenagers benefit from different approaches regarding care and treatment.

Establishing a screening programme for 15-year-olds

In January 1995, a colleague and I set up a pilot scheme within our practice to screen teenagers soon after their fifteenth birthday. We chose this age group because of the timing of the school-leaving booster of diphtheria, tetanus and polio vaccine. It was our intention to evaluate the programme after twelve months.

Main aims and objectives:

- To introduce teenagers to the primary health care team and use of appropriate services provided.
- To encourage uptake of immunisations.
- To make young people aware of lifestyle choices and provide the opportunity to discuss them in a friendly environment.
- To refer to appropriate health services as necessary.

One of the reasons for focusing on this particular group stems from the realisation that unhealthy behaviour at this age has major implications for the future health of the general population. Also, chronic diseases, which are the main cause of mortality in the United Kingdom, often begin silently during childhood and adolescence. Many of these conditions can be prevented, alleviated or delayed through early intervention. *The Health of the Nation* (DoH, 1992) identifies key areas for health promotion, including physical activity, diet, smoking and alcohol misuse, sexual health and accident prevention, all of which are relevant issues for young people. Smoking and poor eating patterns are examples of unhealthy behaviour which can become established during the first twenty years of life. Timely advice at this stage may encourage young people to make changes which will pay dividends in the future, before unhealthy lifestyles become entrenched.

During the planning stage, I located various studies which clearly demonstrate the positive impact that GPs and other members of the primary health care team can make on the health of young people, providing an appropriate health promotion strategy is in place (Donovan and McCarthy, 1988; Hibble and Elwood, 1992; Campbell and Edgar, 1993). It seemed appropriate for community nurses to be involved in this project, as many already possess the appropriate skills to advise and support teenagers regarding their lifestyle choices.

Setting up the clinic

Prior to commencement, discussions took place with the GPs, practice and school nurses, the team leader and the immunisation department. We also enlisted the support of the receptionists and clerks working in the community health office. Fifteen-year-old clients were identified via the practice computer, and sent a personal letter inviting them to attend for an appointment at the surgery soon after their fifteenth birthday. Initially, two health visitors and two school nurses took turns in running the weekly clinic – four teenagers were given 20 minutes for a consultation. Our aim was to provide a dedicated clinic, where a private and confidential discussion could take place within a friendly environment. Previously they would just have been given their booster immunisations during a clinic attended by babies and young children.

During the screening clinic, the young people are given their second booster of low dose diphtheria, tetanus and polio, plus the MMR (measles, mumps and rubella) vaccine, if appropriate. They are weighed, measured and urinalysis is carried out. Blood pressure is also taken and girls are asked about their menstrual history. This information is entered onto their medical records. Any further discussion is confidential, and relevant information will only be shared with their parents or doctor after gaining permission from the individual concerned.

After the clinical procedures have been carried out, the fifteen-year-olds are given the opportunity to discuss lifestyle issues, including diet, exercise, alcohol consumption, smoking, relation-ships, stress and self-esteem. Individual health concerns are also aired, leaflets given where appropriate and referrals made if necessary. In addition, breast awareness is discussed with the girls and testicular examination with the boys.

During the first year, 140 fifteen-year-olds were invited to the clinic and 119 attended (85%), representing a good uptake when compared with other studies. Some of the young people did not attend the clinic, but still received their immunisations with the practice nurses. Altogether 92.5% were immunised, which compared favourably with the Trust figures for this age group (79%). The screening programme seemed to have been well received by both the teenagers and their parents, according to anecdotal evidence. One mother commented that she had been unaware of her daughter's sleeping problems until after she had attended the clinic; having voiced her concerns with the nurse the girl confided with her mother.

In order to evaluate the programme in more depth and improve the service, I decided to find out what the teenagers themselves felt about attending for screening. The following were some of the questions posed:

- ❖ Is the service acceptable? Is it user-friendly?
- ❖ Do the young people feel comfortable?
- ❖ Were the issues discussed relevant to their needs?
- ❖ Are there other health issues, which should be raised?
- ❖ Do the fifteen-year-olds feel they have gained anything by attending?

Evaluation

It seemed appropriate to evaluate the teenage screening clinic as part of my final year research project for a BA (Hons) in Nursing Studies. I was fortunate in receiving valuable support from an experienced supervisor on the university staff. In order to ascertain the feelings of some of the young people who had attended the clinic I carried out a focus group interview with eight teenagers (five girls and three boys) at a local secondary school. Prior to this I had enlisted support from the head teacher and the school nurse, who helped in facilitating the taped discussion.

Detailed findings from this research paper may be found in the unpublished *Evaluation Of A Teenage Screening Programme*, at De Montfort University, Leicester (Freehan, 1996). To summarise, the clinic appeared to be of value to the participating teenagers and most felt that the health issues raised during their consultation had been relevant to their needs. The young people perceived the clinic as an opportunity to have a health MOT, and thought that they should be offered regular appointments.

The study demonstrated that teenagers are individuals, displaying different attitudes towards health issues. Most confessed unhealthy eating habits, and appreciated the need to make improvements in their diets. They wanted expert guidance, backed up by leaflets where necessary. The girls tended to worry about their body image, and appreciated the opportunity to discuss weight and exercise. Smoking and drinking alcohol were also identified as areas of concern for young people, and they said that they wanted more information about drug awareness. Sexual health, as expected, proved a sensitive topic, however there is clearly a need for teenagers to access accurate information from trustworthy sources. This could be a teacher (depending on their knowledge and expertise), although the girls commented that a nurse might be more appropriate for their needs.

As a result of this research, several points were raised to improve the service for fifteen-year-olds:

* compile a health questionnaire for completion, prior to clinic attendance
* provide appropriate health education leaflets in the waiting area
* community staff involved with young people need training and updating in the following areas; substance abuse and drug awareness, nutrition, sexual health and family planning
* adolescents need to be encouraged to make appropriate use of the health services provided, to ensure that they receive relevant information.

In addition, it would be necessary to consider further methods of evaluating the clinic (using questionnaires, for example).

Following this study, a simple health questionnaire was designed and sent to the fifteen-year-olds with an immunisation leaflet and their clinic invitation. This proved a useful tool in sparking discussion on a range of topics. We have also tried to make the consultation more relevant to the young person involved by focusing on their particular health needs. A leaflet rack has been set up with a range of information for young people and their parents. With regard to training, my colleague has attended a course on alcohol awareness, and having undertaken the Diploma in Asthma Care, is a useful source of knowledge in this area. I have accessed training on 'Understanding young people's drug taking', and completed the ENB 901 Family Planning course. We have also developed an information leaflet with a list of telephone numbers and various support services, including specific clinics, which occur within the practice.

The future

I feel a sense of achievement as I have introduced a new initiative at work, which still continues to function effectively four years later. It has often been difficult to find the time to run the clinic, particularly when other responsibilities compete for attention. The two school nurses who started with us in the beginning have left, leaving my health visitor colleague and myself to keep the service operating. Without her sustained commitment and the support of the practice team, particularly the receptionists and the community clerks, we would not have been able to continue the clinics. We have two new school nurses in our area, who have expressed an interest in being involved. Hopefully, they will bring a new dimension to our screening programme, providing an opportunity to examine the service and incorporate fresh ideas.

Clinical supervision has provided a supportive environment to reflect on what we have achieved with teenage screening. Sharing the experience with my peers has enabled me to receive some feedback and draw on the other group members' expertise. Health visitors in neighbouring areas have also initiated screening programmes, which generates further discussion and learning, since others may utilise different approaches in caring for this particular age group.

Tackling a piece of qualitative research has also proved an invaluable experience. Although daunting in the beginning, and time-consuming, the process was both informative and enjoyable. I found out a lot about myself, and the knowledge I gained has been very useful in other aspects of my work.

My colleague and I evaluate the clinic every year, examining attendance, referrals made and topics discussed. We continue to make changes, to improve both the service and organisation of the programme. The percentage of young people attending remains high, and the health issues raised range from diet and weight concerns to skin problems, stress and family planning. Some of the young people have a list of things they wish to address, others just want to complete the process as quickly as possible.

Future possibilities include expanding the clinic beyond the GP practice, to meet the needs of other young people in the locality. Teenagers could be offered a range of services including dietary advice, support while trying to stop smoking, counselling and sexual health services. There is tremendous scope for development. However, any youth project needs to be approached with tact and sensitivity, particularly regarding family planning issues, and the support of the community is paramount. Working with young people can be challenging and rewarding, especially when one is able to advise and help an individual who feels secure enough to share his/her concerns for the first time.

My role as a health visitor continues to develop, and will possibly change again when primary care groups begin to make an impact. Fortunately the work is varied, and never boring, and I feel privileged in having the opportunity to carry out health promotion with young people. Health visitors are keen to demonstrate that their responsibilities extend beyond the child under five, and this initiative has given me scope to develop my skills.

Key questions and discussion points

- ❖ Is there a need for this sort of adolescent health screening to be more freely available to all concerned?
- ❖ Is June reaching the client group most at need?
- ❖ What are the difficulties in maintaining this sort of practice development on an ongoing basis, where immediate hard outcome data is not available?

10.

Looking inside endoscopy

Bernice Litchfield

Bernice Litchfield RGN is currently working as a nurse endoscopist within the gastrointestinal department of a large city hospital.

❖ This account looks at the change required to extend the nurse's role and push out the barriers of nursing practice.

The word endoscopy comes from the Greek 'to examine within'. The function of an endoscopy is to render the interior of a cavity observable to the endoscopist as if it were being viewed directly. Over a period of about one hundred and fifty years, people experimented with tubes and light trying to develop the endoscope.

In 1806 Bozzini discovered that it was possible to look inside selected organs with a hollow rigid tube and a candle. Kelling (1897) designed a rigid gastroscope, the lower third of which was flexible to 40 degrees, supplying light with a miniature electric globe and a prism. Schindler (1936) completed the second phase of the flexible gastroscope by adding lenses, air channels, electric connection and an eye piece. He supplied light using prisms, lenses and an electric globe. In 1930 Lamm demonstrated that fine glass fibre threads, bundled together and angled, could be used to produce and direct light, but this was not developed for decades.

Hirschowitz in 1958 produced the first flexible oesophago-gastroduodenosope (gastroscope) which gave the required views and enabled photographs to be taken. Modern technology has allowed flexible endoscopes to be further improved enabling endoscopists to provide a comprehensive diagnostic and therapeutic endoscopy service.

In the 1970s flexible gastroscopes were used mainly by the surgeons to detect duodenal ulcers, greatly reducing the demand for diagnosing by laparotomy. Endoscopy was the way forward. A seminar room in a surgical day care ward was altered to allow selected surgical and medical doctors to provide an endoscopy service while a purpose built endoscopy unit was designed, funded and finally built.

In 1987 I started working, first as an enrolled nurse then as a staff nurse, in endoscopy on the surgical day care ward, where I developed patient documentation and information leaflets and competency based teaching packages for endoscopy nursing staff.

These aimed to ensure a safe, friendly, relaxed atmosphere in which patients could have their endoscopic procedures performed. The new endoscopy unit opened in 1993 and became evident that the demand for endoscopy was outstripping the available service. Nurse endoscopy was proposed to provide a continuing service for patients.

After supervision and training I officially started my job as nurse endoscopist on 1 October, 1996. I had several concerns about the role. How would medical staff, who had previously performed the procedures I was now performing, react towards me? How would I gain the confidence of general practitioners who had already whispered that a second class service would be provided by a nurse? My own legal cover. I would not be able to cope with the workload of endoscoping and continuing other nursing duties which still had to continue to enable the unit to function efficiently.

A typical day

A typical day starts at 8.00 am. The unit is opened and the emergency wards contacted to see if they have any patients with gastrointestinal bleeding.

Clinic areas, endoscopy rooms and the recovery area are prepared ensuring all necessary equipment needed is available and in working order. I familiarise myself with the history of patients attending for procedures on my endoscopy list.

Patients arriving in the endoscopy room for their procedure, are greeted warmly and introduced to myself and the other members of staff in the room. I answer any questions they may have before asking them to sign their consent form, after which they are suitably positioned on the examination couch. Pulse oximetry and oxygen saturation are monitored throughout the procedure. If sedation is required, intravenous access is gained with a venflon and sedation given in accordance with the sedation protocol and the Trust's intravenous drug administration policy .

Post procedure the patient is recovered by a trained person who reports any untoward occurrences immediately to me. When fully recovered I give all necessary explanations regarding the procedure, health education, advice, and information about follow-up, or they are seen by the doctor, depending on the type of list/clinic taking place.

Strategic/operational difficulties encountered and resolutions

For nurse endoscopy to take place at my employing Trust, certain criteria had to be addressed:

- ❖ The Trust Board had to give approval and accept liability.
- ❖ The consultant gastroenterologist had to accept overall responsibility of the nurse endoscopist.
- ❖ Protocols had to be developed to cover patient selection and to carry out procedures with a defined level of supervision.
- ❖ Audit and quality monitoring by a specialist registrar/ consultant endoscopist.
- ❖ A risk management system to identify potential problems had to be instigated.
- ❖ A nurse training programme, including competencies and assessment criteria, had to be introduced.

Senior nursing and medical staff discussed these proposals with the hospital Trust Board members.

To ensure safety during nurse endoscopy lists, a specialist registrar or consultant is required to be on the endoscopy unit at all times.

The endoscopy unit is situated in a new building of the hospital's ever growing complex. Surgical and medical outpatient clinics were located in the older buildings which made them even further away from the procedural area. This created more problems for patients having to find their way to two if not three locations. This was resolved by re-designing the endoscopy unit to enable all endoscopic procedures lists and clinics to be centralised onto the endoscopy unit. With careful planning of these medical and surgical clinics and endoscopy lists, it is possible to always have either a specialist registrar or consultant on the unit (1999).

Before my endoscopy training could begin I addressed some basic additional skill requirements. Having a fear of needles made learning to venepuncture and cannulate somewhat traumatic. I attended study days to be competent at giving intravenous drugs, and became proficient at advanced life support. I increased my understanding relating to accountability and autonomous practice; legal and ethical issues relating to taking on this role; the nurse's role in promoting health education; being aware of and being able to apply evidence-based practice; evaluating practice using audit.

I was very conscious that to fulfil all these criteria would be demanding not only on me but on the other endoscopy staff in the unit. We worked together as a team, through the re-designing of the unit and my training programme, and maintained an effective endoscopy service throughout.

Traditionally only doctors endoscoped at the Trust assisted mainly by qualified nursing staff. While planning the service redesign, an analysis of nursing activity was carried out, which showed qualified nursing staff spent only two per cent of their time in direct nursing care with the remainder of the time spent in departmental administration and the maintenance of equipment.

The word 'qualified' was exchanged for the word 'trained' and appropriately trained persons, 'team associates', were employed. All necessary training was given once they were in post. The number of qualified nurses in the unit was reduced. Once the team associates were competency trained by the nursing staff in all aspects of endoscopy work, they were able to act as first assistants to both medical and nurse endoscopists.

As many of the patients passing through our unit require venepuncture or cannulation or both, these two procedures have become second nature to me, but I know I would not have persevered and mastered this phobia without the continual words of encouragement and support from my colleagues.

Permission from some consultants to enable nurses to sedate their patients requiring endoscopic procedures was not always given in the early stages of nurse endoscopy, as they still considered it to be the role of junior doctors. As their training programmes became more specialised, reducing the availability of junior doctors to provide a high quality continuing service, nurse endoscopy was viewed as the way forward and gained acknowledgement from these consultants.

With the introduction of *The Patient's Charter* (DoH, 1991), patients were becoming used to nurse led clinics and in many cases preferred nurses to perform procedures. After successful completion of my training, nurse endoscopy lists became more available.

Audit has shown the development of the role of nurse endoscopy provides a patient focused, high quality, fast response service in a radically redesigned service.

In an Open Day for GPs where they attended the gastro-enterology centre and observed while I endoscoped patients, they saw that their referred patients were receiving a very high quality service. Photographs and routine biopsies are taken in most nurse endoscopy procedures and more serious findings are viewed by a senior doctor within minutes and appropriate action taken.

Working alongside medical colleagues and performing diagnostic procedures for patients on their first, and often, only visit to the hospital give considerable job satisfaction.

Audit shows that two thirds of all diagnostic work is performed on nurse endoscopy lists. Waiting lists have been radically reduced from a few months to a few weeks.

In the future, nurse endoscopy may develop to incorporate selected therapeutic procedures. Some areas have been identified but risk management and protocols have not been completed. It is hoped that consultants will continue to be as encouraging with these future developments as they have been in the initial stages of nurse endoscopy. I am sure that by working together in a multi-disciplinary team we will continue to provide a high quality service at the Leicester Royal Infirmary to keep us at the forefront of patient care.

Key questions and discussion points

❖ Bernice describes how an innovative nursing role developed because the workload of medical staff was developing beyond their resources. Is this true of other practice developments that have occurred?

❖ Has the quality of service received by the patients increased or decreased? On what criteria do you base your answer?

❖ Are there areas within your own speciality where similar developments could take place? If so, what is preventing them from occurring?

11.

A reflective account of practice development

Alison Wells

Alison Wells RGN, RM Dip. N Dip Ed, BA (Hons) currently works as change manager within a centre of best practice in a large city hospital.

❖ This account describes the joys and frustrations of working as a clinical educator in a large medical unit of a busy inner city hospital.

Training and development of professional and clinical skills at the Leicester Royal Infirmary take place in each of the eight clinical directorates. Each directorate employs a clinical educator whose hours of work differ according to the size of the directorate. The medical directorate is the largest directorate and employs a colleague and myself on a full-time basis. I am responsible for the training budget; we share other tasks according to our abilities, availability and preference.

My colleague and I have different but complementary skills and so we work very well together. Our responsibilities include the training and development of all staff within the directorate (administrative and clerical staff, medical staff and nurses). We deliver training on clinical skills (phlebotomy, cannulation, intravenous drug administration, etc). We also provide support with profiling, clinical supervision and other professional issues. Coaching teams from wards and departments takes up a great deal of our time. We take teams out for the day to help them develop and identify areas for change.

The role also incorporates activities at a strategic level, ranging from influencing and developing policies to providing professional advice to non nurses. A training and development post had existed for some time before I was appointed. I completed a full-time teaching course and was seconded into the role. I was later employed on a permanent basis following re-organisation of the directorate.

Initially I felt excited about the post, but was concerned about whether I could do it. I recall at the start of the secondment, sitting in the office with a blank diary wondering where on earth to start. It was strange not having someone else dictate your activities for the day (drugs at eight, ward round at ten, bed baths in between). My other concern was gaining credibilty with all the staff in the directorate (over 400 people). It was also strange to be able to drink coffee while I worked, something you definitely could not do on the ward.

A typical day

I arrive at work at about eight in the morning (in order to miss the traffic and find a parking space). Meetings do not generally start until nine and clinical staff are usually very busy at this time, so this gives me an opportunity to catch up on paperwork and my mail (electronic and paper).

On a typical day I will probably attend a meeting, this could be with the managers in the Directorate or with colleagues in similar posts across the hospital. Clinical staff who want to develop some training in their area also meet with me to discuss their ideas.

I also act as clinical supervisor to several people and so may have an hour put aside to meet one of them. I may also have a session arranged with a group of nursing auxiliaries whom I support my colleague in supervising.

The time out days we facilitate take a lot of preparation, from organising the activities to booking venues and sending out invitations. Often these days can be quite sensitive, particularly if medical staff are involved, as they do not like playing games! Some days can feel as if I have achieved very little, staff often pop in for advice, support or just a cup of coffee. This is something we have encouraged but it can mean that any work I have planned, I do not complete. I sometimes work through lunch but do try to get out of the office as often as possible. A group of us (my colleagues, some of the managers and myself) often meets up in the staff canteen.

I sometimes teach, and on a typical day will have a session to deliver. My favourite is, What's going on? During these sessions the participants vote on what they want to discuss. I arrange to have experts on standby, as anything can come up, from clinical governance to the forthcoming hospital merger.

As the training and development budget holder I have to make decisions about funding for courses and study days. This is one of my least favourite jobs as I am not terribly effective at managing money. My other responsibility is to collate the Education Consortia requirements for the directorate. This is my pet hate as it is difficult to predict our requirements for the future, so we never get it quite right.

I usually finish work at about five o'clock. I rarely take things home to do other than perhaps some reading and maybe a bit of shopping for equipment for the time out days. The first couple of years in the role presented me with a few difficulties. I have already discussed my concern about my credibility, which I had initially felt would be an issue with ward staff but it arose with other staff groups too.

I also had to gain credibility with managers and doctors. Achieving credibility with nurses was the least of my problems in reality. I worked on each of the wards for the first few months in post to demonstrate my clinical ability and my willingness to wipe bottoms.

The managers were more difficult. They didn't understand the role, or at least had a different understanding of the role to mine. Initially, training and development were not an integral part of the directorate but were viewed as an add-on. The function of training and development was about delivering mandatory training and getting nurses equipped to administer intravenous drugs as soon as possible. Not everyone recognised that training and development were a fundamental part of a good organisation.

Other difficulties I encountered were achieving a balance between directorate work and strategic work, the problem of measuring outcomes and the scope of the role.

In order to gain credibility with the managers, I started to attend their meetings even if there was nothing of direct relevance to my role on the agenda. I tried to contribute as much as possible and found I had quite a lot to offer as an objective onlooker. I became an accepted member of the team, and training and development are now often on the agenda. I went on to develop a strategy for training and development for the directorate that linked to the Trust strategy

This added some weight and credence to the role and it is now updated annually.

Gaining credibility with the medical staff is a whole different ball game; I am not sure I've succeeded yet. My colleague delivers training to medical students, but we have yet to gain access into teaching qualified doctors.

Measuring outcomes is extremely difficult, but unfortunately something that my manager demanded. We can provide figures that demonstrate 'bums on seats' but measuring learning outcomes is not as straight forward. I feel that the only way to demonstrate success is time. Eventually long term projects come to fruition, staff go back to managers and give positive feedback about training they've attended and sooner or later the training and development team gains a good reputation. This is frustrating, particularly for business managers who want hard facts and figures.

Reflection

In the second year of my role, I had a new line manager. I was still relatively unsure of the role, but was gaining confidence in certain aspects. My first appraisal with my manager started well. I had prepared my objectives carefully. These reflected my personal development needs and what I anticipated would be the needs of the directorate. I was unsure of what my manager would want and I am sure she was unsure of what to expect from me.

My manager raised concerns about the amount of time I spent working in trust wide forums and about the amount of 'hands on' care I delivered. These two areas have and still do provide me with dilemmas. I felt it was important for me to represent the directorate on trust wide forums. I was able to influence decision-making at a fairly high level and made the most of the opportunities to do so. The work carried out in these forums can often be fairly slow, while members attempt to reach a consensus. However, sooner or later the work accomplished impacts on the activities in the directorate. I wanted to ensure that this had a positive benefit to the directorate and to nurses.

An example is the intravenous drug administration policy and training package. Both took many hours to complete. Some directorates' had their own training packages (including the medical directorate) and others accessed the medical directorate training sessions. This had implications, different standards of training were delivered and the medical directorate picked up other directorates' work. This was sometimes at the expense of its own staff. Once completed, the new package that was competency and evidence-based was delivered by all clinical educators to staff from different directorates. The package is reviewed annually. The benefits to the directorate were that the package was more comprehensive and up-to-date. There were more sessions available that staff could attend and they worked in groups that comprised of staff from all over the hospital. From the clinical educators' point of view, they had fewer sessions to deliver, so reducing their workload.

The second issue, the amount of time I spent delivering care, also caused me considerable anxiety and continues to do so. As I have already said, I spent time on each of the wards during the first few weeks in post in order to gain clinical credibility. However, I found it difficult to continue to do this on a regular basis.

Practice development is a broad remit and it is hard to manage your time and prioritise activities. It is also the kind of job that grows as you become more experienced and confident. Clinical credibility is vital. I found that when I worked on the wards, people were dubious about my motives, was I checking on them? How much was I being paid to work as an 'E' grade staff nurse? Was I reporting my findings to their manager? I had forgotten what it was like when the senior nurse (or matron) came to help, it was terrifying. Unless I had clear objectives for being there, I was viewed with suspicion.

In response to my manager's concerns, I agreed to increase my activities within the directorate and spend more time in the clinical areas.

So, while my manager was wise to be concerned about these two issues, her anxiety unsettled me. I felt angry that she should question my judgement, frustrated because I thought that I knew what I was doing and worried that I might not be able to meet her expectations. I resented (unjustifiably, I realise now) my manager's interference with my work. I felt my manager was questioning the value of the role.

The good things about the experience were that it enabled both of us to clarify our expectations of training and development. It made me much more aware of how I spent my time. I worked harder, trying to pull everything in so that I could do what I wanted and achieve my objectives. Nevertheless, I was less open with my manager for a while and continued to work in a way that I thought was appropriate. I spent half, not full days, on the wards. I continued to work in trust wide forums, ironically gaining credibility among my peers and with managers outside the directorate.

At my appraisal a year later, my manager was pleased with my progress. She had heard about the work I was achieving in Trust forums and acknowledged that this work was worthwhile. I discussed openly and honestly my struggle to work clinically and how this caused conflict with my other activities. It had by this time also started to niggle at my conscience, as wards became short-staffed and activity increased. It was agreed that I should join the nursing bank (my suggestion). I continue to do this. The benefits are that I am paid as a staff nurse, I keep myself updated and I do not have to juggle my workload with clinical work. Above all, I maintain some credibility. The benefits to the directorate are that they use me when they most need me and pay me according to the work I do. The staff also seem less threatened by my presence when they are understaffed.

On reflection, I can see that my manager had little knowledge of my ability and faced the same challenges that I did: meeting objectives and gaining credibility. She had to justify employing a nurse on a senior grade to deliver training and development and she needed to see some impact and measurable outcomes. Robbins and Finley (1998) discuss the importance of trust in teams. It is a two-way process with leaders having to trust team members and vice versa. In hindsight it is understandable that my manager and I faced this conflict.

Since this incident, I have encountered a number of people in similar roles who face similar conflicts. Should a similar situation arise again, I would not agree to objectives I was not confident in achieving. If unable to meet an agreement, I would ask for some time to think about the objectives and then arrange to meet with my manager again. I would hope that both of us would have time to consider both sides of the argument and agree a compromise. I would take the challenge to my role less personally and recognise that I might have a better understanding of the role, but must be willing to prove this.

Key questions and discussion points

❖ Alison identifies an increasingly common experience of a job that combines a number of separate roles, teacher, administrator, clinician, manager, researcher etc. How can we achieve an appropriate balance and not become overloaded by the potential volume of work?

❖ Alison demonstrates that not only do we have to do the job, but to produce the evidence in terms of measurable outcomes that we have done the job. What are the difficulties in achieving both, without the activity compromising your role?

❖ What possible solutions are there to the agenda conflict of managers and practice development staff?

❖ A number of jobs like these can pull us in various directions. How can we get and give support to people in these and similar roles?

12.

Teaching consultation skills to medical students

Adrian Hastings

Adrian Hastings MB Ch B is a teaching co-ordinator at the Department of General Practice and Primary Health Care, University of Leicester and a partner in a busy GP practice.

❖ Adrian describes this unusual role and reflects upon the assessment model that has been developed for medical students.

The work of a lecturer practitioner GP

The course, the students and their teachers

Those of us who work in undergraduate medical education are fortunate. Compared with most other university departments the resources available for teaching are generous, and the quality of applicants for places on our courses is high. We would be able to fill our courses two or three times over with young people with the ability to become good doctors. Despite this, successive committees which have looked at medical education, have criticised the emphasis placed on acquiring factual knowledge and overcrowding of the curriculum with subjects more appropriately learnt after graduation (Todd, 1968; Merrison, 1975). The most recent report *Tomorrow's Doctors* by the General Medical Council drew attention to the failure of previous attempts to radically reform medical education (GMC, 1993). It made a series of recommendations that have helped to modernise curricula in most UK medical schools. The GMC recommended a reduction in the burden of factual information and the adoption of learning through curiosity with the capacity for self-education. The importance of teaching essential skills and inculcating appropriate attitudes was highlighted. The GMC believed that the core curriculum should be based on body systems (eg. respiratory system), with basic scientists and clinicians integrating their contributions to common purpose, thus eliminating the rigid pre-clinical/clinical division of traditional medical education. The

78

report acknowledged that there was a need for more of the curriculum to be delivered in primary care and other community settings. It also recommended that systems of assessment should be adopted which were appropriate to a student centred learning style and which examined, in particular, the core clinical skills of history taking, examination, problem-solving and patient management. It was against this background that I became the teaching co-ordinator in the Department of General Practice and Primary Health Care at the University of Leicester.

I divide my time equally between my practice as a GP in a busy inner city practice and as a lecturer in a university department.

A typical working day at the university will entail administration, teaching, course development and evaluation and sometimes opportunities for research. The main course taught by the department is in clinical methods. In small groups (seven to nine) we aim to provide our students with the theoretical background to their learning in general practice and hospital settings. This enables them to understand how doctors reach diagnoses and what information they need to gather from patients to decide on the nature of the problem. We encourage them to adopt a patient-centred consultation style. They are also asked to consider how to manage presenting problems and negotiate this management with patients. In departmental teaching we use a variety of techniques, including small group instruction, case analysis, video taped consultations and group work with simulated patients, including sessions on how to break bad news. At an earlier stage in the curriculum we teach basic communication skills through role-play with simulated patients. We also arrange for students to visit families where there is significant chronic illness to learn more about the physical, social and psychological consequences of illness, so that they adopt a holistic approach to their patients. It is my personal responsibility to ensure that the administration of the teaching programme is efficient. As this involves the placement of 180 students each year to 50 different practices and three hospitals this is no mean task. I have to ensure that the quality of the teaching in the different settings is good and that all the teachers understand the course objectives. I also organise the practice-based end-point assessment, which takes half a day for each student and involves two general practice assessors.

Aspirations and obstacles

The clinical methods course occupies an eight-week block half way through the medical course (Hastings *et al*, in press). By this time students have a considerable amount of knowledge and the basic clinical skills of history taking and physical examination. What they struggle with, at this stage in their professional development, is the integration of knowledge with skills to problem-solve patients' complaints. The course concentrates on development of their consultation performance and is integrated into the overall curriculum because it further develops skills they have acquired previously. We chose to teach students simultaneously in practice and hospital settings so they could understand that the core clinical skills of all doctors are the same, regardless of where they are exercised.

When I started co-ordinating the clinical methods course, I hoped that students would feel the course had been a pivotal point in their professional development, and that they would understand the consultation better and be more able to conduct it well. We expected that practice-based clinical teachers, who had a tradition of teaching a similar course, would be able to grasp the aims and objectives of the new course quickly. We believed that they would provide students with many opportunities to consult with patients and give immediate feedback on the performance.

My fear was that there would be insufficient resources to buy the protected time of general practitioners to do the teaching. We were also concerned that hospital teachers would feel uneasy with teaching consultation skills and would prefer to emphasise the acquisition of factual knowledge.

If the future of undergraduate medical education is to match the GMC's intentions it will be necessary to overcome some important strategic obstacles. Medical teachers have to make a conceptual jump in their thinking about education. There has been a strong tradition to value the acquisition of detailed knowledge over that of skills. Assessment in medical education has relied heavily on factual tests such as multiple-choice questions, which are poor predictors of clinical performance (Johnson and Reynard, 1994). The majority of medical teachers that students encounter are highly knowledgeable in a narrow field and find it difficult to judge the degree of knowledge students require in their particular discipline. The teaching of skills such as good communication is often seen as a 'bolt on' addition done by GPs or psychologists, rather than an essential attribute of all doctors that should be taught well by all doctors.

Modern medical curricula are delivered in modules and blocks of clinical attachments. Two or three hundred different people will teach each student during their undergraduate career. Each module has its own assessment and there is a tendency for students to pass from one to the other without teachers in the next block building on from the previous learning. Insight into a student's learning needs, which might have taken one teacher several weeks to gain, are therefore lost and have to be rediscovered by subsequent teachers.

A major obstacle to developing consultation skills is the high proportion of teaching sessions that are passive. Students frequently complain of observing qualified doctors at work without being actively involved (Hastings *et al*, in press). Because of the pressure of clinical work, and because some clinical teachers are conscripts rather than volunteers, teaching sessions are often not delivered. Teachers may only have a vague awareness of the objectives of the course and therefore fall back on their own experiences to help them decide what to teach. Furthermore, practising clinicians have rarely undergone any professional training in teaching and are not familiar with current thinking on which methods are most effective. Although medical students encounter many gifted, instinctive teachers, there are still all too many enthusiastic practitioners of 'teaching by terror' as practised by Lancelot Sprat in the *Doctor in the House* films.

Although tests of knowledge such as MCQ papers can help a learner assess their grasp of essential facts, they are not useful in summative assessment. They are reliable and welcomed by teachers because they are easy to mark. However there is no evidence that those students who perform well in knowledge tests are able to use their knowledge in clinical problem-solving or are better able to relate to patients (Tutton, 1996; Lynch *et al*, 1998). More sophisticated written examinations, such as short essay papers, are a better test of ability to apply knowledge in specific contexts.

However, these still do not predict performance across the range of complex professional skills such as those required by a doctor. If we have a reliable instrument to assess consultation performance in summative assessment, then we can safely abandon the quest for reliable and valid knowledge tests. Provided a sufficient sample of consultations is observed, it is impossible for a student to demonstrate good interviewing and problem-solving skills and to develop holistic management plans of patients' problems without a sound grounding of clinical knowledge.

It is generally believed that 'assessment drives the learning'. If we accept this, then the only logical way to assess student consultation performance must be to observe them consulting with patients. Such assessments are labour intensive as they have to be conducted in real time, and if the assessment is to be summative then two assessors are required to ensure reliability and equity. In order for the assessment to be valid the assessors must use criteria that are well understood by the student and the assessors. As observation of clinical practice involves a considerable element of professional judgement the assessors will require careful training to ensure that they make similar judgements of the same observed performance.

Successes and future opportunities

We use the Leicester Assessment Package (LAP) to judge the consultation performance of medical undergraduates. It was developed from a similar instrument designed to test the consultation performance of general practitioners (Fraser *et al*, 1994a). Students are assessed in five categories of consultation performance:

+ interviewing and history taking
+ physical examination
+ patient management
+ problem-solving
+ behaviour and relationship with patients.

The necessary skills in each category are further broken down into a series of competencies. The package includes criteria to define different levels of performance, which are graded on a six-point scale when the instrument is being used in summative assessment. At the end of an eight-week course in clinical methods a pair of general practitioners, one of whom is external to the practice and has undergone further training, assesses students. They observe the student consulting with five patients. The patients are not pre-selected except that the reception staff are asked to book new patient problems as far as practical. The assessment is carried out in a GP consulting room and the student is required to see five patients within two hours, although the time each consultation lasts is dependent on the complexity of the problem. At the time of writing over 350 students have been assessed using 1750 patients.

The patients are drawn from the whole age range and include those with minor illness through to the first presentation of cancer or severe depression. At the end of the consultation the student leaves the room and the patient's own doctor completes the consultation. Sometimes this is simply a matter of affirming the student's diagnosis and management. At other times the doctor may need to re-run the consultation and end with a different conclusion.

After the observation phase of the assessment the two assessors independently award a grade and then confer to decide the student's strengths and areas requiring improvement. This process usually takes about an hour. Giving oral feedback, using the process described by Pendleton completes the assessment (Pendleton *et al*, 1984). A written report is prepared which is then sent to the student. This not only describes the strengths and areas requiring improvement identified by the assessment, but also includes specific strategies to help the student improve.

The logistics of such a process are formidable. Each assessment takes seven hours of assessor time. As most of the external assessors are members of the department and 175 students are assessed each year this is a significant call on the time of clinical lecturers. How can this investment in time be justified?

In order for an assessment to be a good one it must have five attributes: validity; reliability; acceptability; feasibility; educational impact. We are unaware of a more valid way of assessing a student's consultation performance than direct observation. In order to ensure the assessment is reliable, it is necessary to demonstrate that two independent observers are likely to reach a similar conclusion when they observe the same performance. Earlier work has established the reliability of the LAP (Fraser *et al*, 1994b). Experience in using it for the first two years has shown it produces highly reliable judgements about students on the pass/fail boundary, and sufficiently reliable results for the numerical mark for all students. The reliability is comparable to any other assessment tool and better than many. Every student at the end of their assessment is asked to complete a feedback questionnaire with 15 questions about the assessment and feedback process. Students consistently award very high scores (in excess of four on a scale where five is the maximum) to all aspects of the process (McKinley, Fraser, van de Vleuten, in press). Is the method of assessment acceptable to patients? We have not evaluated this formally, but there have been no instances of complaints about students by any of the patients involved. Patients often comment favourably about the students and say that they appreciate the extra information they learn when students explain their diagnostic reasoning and reasons for choosing their management plan. The fact that we have delivered this assessment process on 350 occasions and that we intend to continue to do so shows that in our view it is feasible. What is the educational impact? We have asked the students, six months after completing their course, how useful they found the assessment and feedback they were given.

Although the appreciation scores have declined in the intervening period — as expected given they were so high in the first place — they still express high levels of appreciation of both the process and feedback they were given. In addition, summative assessments that students undergo prior to entering the final phase of their course and in their finals examination use a similar process. These assessments are conducted in hospital, using hospital patients and so students do perceive some differences in the process. However, Leicester students receive a very clear message that the medical school requires, above all else, that they are effective in consulting with patients.

As this is the key professional skill that virtually all doctors require throughout their professional career, it is gratifying to know that our assessment methods encourage students to consult well with patients.

The accuracy of any measurement instrument depends to some degree on the person using it. Assessing complex consultation skills requires a considerable element of professional judgement and many facets have to be assessed. Therefore, for even a good tool with demonstrated reliability to work well, assessors require careful preparation. Every assessor has to complete four days of training before they can undertake an end of course assessment. After instruction and practice in using the LAP to analyse video-taped consultations, current students volunteer to be observed consulting with simulated patients, and to receive feedback from clinical teachers attending the training workshops (Preston-Whyte *et al*, 1993). The training encompasses making a judgement of performance and the preparation of written and oral feedback.

Compiling 350 assessment reports has given us the opportunity to identify the principal strengths of medical undergraduates at this stage in their career and how to help them improve. Many students have difficulty in accessing the knowledge they hold. They have learnt many facts about diseases and the working of body systems. However, this knowledge is held in different areas in their minds and they have trouble in linking the information they gather from patients with their theoretical knowledge to solve the problem. Medical students commonly demonstrate lack of awareness of the social and psychological factors affecting both the presentation of physical disease and its management. They are taught to ask why patients have come to the doctor, and to discover their ideas, concerns and expectations of the consultation, but often have difficulty in doing this in a manner that encourages patients to open up about their fears. Although students complain that we ask them to diagnose and manage problems about which they have insufficient knowledge, the reality is usually a deficiency of skills.

The strategies that we give them to overcome weaknesses are specific and focused to the problems they have displayed during the assessment. The intention is that they are practical and easily applied in other clinical settings. The following are a selection of those we offer to overcome weaknesses in the interviewing of patients:

- start with open statements, eg. 'Tell me in your own words about the pain'
- demonstrate to the patient that you are listening, eg. by eye contact and nodding
- try to tolerate the discomfort of appropriate silences
- elicit the patient's ideas, concerns and expectations in every consultation
- when satisfied that physical disease is present, always consider its impact on the social and psychological well-being of the patient.

To help them access facts buried in their memories, we encourage them to think through the problem using their basic clinical knowledge. For example, if presented with a young, female patient with lower abdominal pain they may complain, 'I have not done gynaecology yet'. We then ask them to recall the anatomy of the female genital tract and their knowledge of different types of diseases (infection, neoplasm, degenerative etc.) which might affect it. Once they have thought about these they are usually able to work through the clinical problem.

It is very satisfying that analysis of the independent scores by pairs of assessors, shows that this method of assessment makes reliable judgements, particularly of students who may be unsatisfactory (McKinley and Fraser, van de Vleuten, in press). Students consider it to be fair and valid and feel the strategies we give them on how to improve will be of use. As a result of carrying out these assessments we have developed a rich insight into the strengths and weaknesses of Leicester undergraduates at this stage in their career. These could greatly improve the medical course if they are fed back into curriculum design and teacher preparation. If all clinicians responsible for teaching clinical skills were aware of the general needs of students and the particular needs of individuals, this would have a beneficial effect on their teaching.

Although this assessment process is detailed there is still much scope for improving the quality of both the oral and written feedback. We know that students appreciate it but subsequent follow up suggests that the opportunities for using their feedback are limited by the lack of awareness of other teachers on how to incorporate these strategies into their teaching. Although the process is reliable it is important to widen the pool of assessors to include hospital teachers as well as general practitioners. Further training in how to write and deliver feedback to students would help to improve the process greatly.

If this method of improving consultation performance of medical students is the best available it should be possible to adapt for use in other settings. We are currently developing a version of the LAP to analyse consultations by primary care nurses with patients. There are many features of these consultations that are common between doctors and nurses. However, our main interest is to develop an educational tool rather than an assessment instrument as the professional development of nurses is assessed in other ways.

The problems students have with the integration of their learning as the curriculum unfolds must be addressed. At the start I alluded to the relative richness of resources medical educators have available to them. Therefore it is incumbent upon us to provide students with the highest quality learning experiences. I liken the medical curriculum to a series of closed rooms in an art gallery. When visitors enter each new room the curators tell them about the pictures on the wall in that room but have no curiosity about their previous knowledge of art and how it can help understand human nature. How much faster would the visitor learn and understand if the curators built upon their previous experiences?

I have learnt much from helping to develop the assessment of consultation skills of medical students. It is important to be able to break a complex task down into small components to analyse it and to teach it. Everyone can recognise a good consultation compared with a bad one – but it is much harder to move from 'That was good' to, 'the patient was very satisfied because…', and give three key reasons why it went well. Helping students to tap into their prior knowledge is much more rewarding than delivering facts for them to remember – especially when you know the student has studied these very facts before. Skills can only be taught and learnt by observing practice and providing specific strategies about how to improve – exhortations to 'read more' or 'learn a list' only result in further impediments to intelligent thought. More importantly, I have understood that direct measures are vastly superior to proxy ones. If you want to know who is a good doctor – watch them at work. Do not expect exam results, an impressive list of courses attended or testimonials from colleagues (who may be friends) to give you the same answer.

Key questions and discussion points

❖ Adrian states that each student will be taught by several hundred different people throughout their training. How does this compare to your profession?

❖ The assessment model that Adrian describes is time-consuming and administratively complex. Do you as a potential patient feel it is a good system. If so, on what are you basing your judgement.

❖ In what way is this system developing practice?

13.

Baking a cake, nursing style

Jonathan Carver

Jonathan Carver RGN, BSc (Hons,) ENB Higher Award, ENB 124, Cert
Health Ed works as a lecturer practitioner specialising in cardiac nursing.

❖ Jonathan has a joint appointment as a lecturer practitioner in cardiac
nursing. His job description has an overriding aim of fostering
research mindedness.

❖ Jonathan uses a culinary analogy to highlight his varied lecturer
practitioner role.

Providing an overview of your job or role is a bit like describing the
ingredients and experiences of baking a cake. You take a little bit of
this and a little bit of that, all in appropriate measures, and mix. Once
the consistency is right and you have pre-heated your oven, you cook
the mixture to create a new and enjoyable product. Well, that is the
plan.

I do not feel I have reached the end product yet, but I have been in
a few hot kitchens and I have burnt my fingers a few times. My cakes
do not yet have all the necessary ingredients. However, the basic
ingredients are there, they just need a little bit of coaxing and
adaptation.

My main ingredient and thus my hot kitchen, is the clinical
environment of coronary care. My present role is Charge Nurse in a
regional cardiac centre, here in Leicester. I work in a four-bed
coronary care unit (CCU) and a combined 21-bed cardiology ward. I
have been in this post for three years and it has provided me with a
variety of unique opportunities to expand my role and develop my
clinical skills. My day-to-day role on the unit or ward is, I am sure,
typical of most acute areas. It is busy, it is noisy and it can be very
rewarding as well as frustrating. I normally have responsibility for
the shift, frequently covering the rest of the cardiology unit as the
senior nurse on duty. I also act as mentor to a number of students,
both pre and post registration, which provides a separate challenge
from the management of the ward. The area receives patients from
across the Trent region, providing a variety of acute and chronic
cardiac conditions that require adaptability and flexibility from the
staff in managing their caseload.

The area is continually involved with research, frequently at the cutting edge of treatment and, as such, requires continuous consideration for practice changes and the impact of treatment on patients and clients. Further, this continuing, changing environment often presents opportunities for the development of skills that are useful and pertinent to the support of patient care.

My time in this clinical environment has resulted in the acquisition of skills in: ECG (electrocardiograph) recording and interpretation; phlebotomy and cannulation; basic and advanced life support provision and training, including the administration of first line drugs used in cardiac arrest; arterial sheath removal; health education.

These skills allow for the provision of a more holistic approach to care management, although the catalyst for acquiring such roles should be patient focused rather than medically led (Carver, 1998). I use these roles on a daily basis to support both patient care and the development of colleagues and students. However, two key factors in the acquisition of these skills are knowledge and experience. Without experience and reflecting on that experience, it would be difficult to analyse and adapt these roles in the right circumstances at the right time. As such, experience supports tacit knowledge, where what I know and what I experience are critically linked through reflection. Further, my analysis of these roles in practice is based on their effectiveness and promotion of care delivery.

The acquisition of these types of skills provides a depth and breadth of knowledge that can be integrated into patient care and staff development. I can act as a role model, using these skills to present a professional and efficient model of care. This skill acquisition also provides opportunities to act in a more holistic manner for my patients. Managing care with these skills has been suggested to enhance patient care (Carver, 1998), as the relationship between patient and nurse develops with the greater time spent by one nurse with one patient.

This clinical background also provides a number of learning opportunities for students, and requires all staff to be adaptable in their facilitation of learners, whether pre or post registration. The skills and knowledge I have developed, alongside my enthusiasm for facilitating learning, resulted in a move into a more formal teaching situation over the last year and I presently lead two modules on a degree course for the BSc Health Studies/ENB 254 (cardiac nursing) programme through De Montfort University. Thus my role is one of clinical 'expert' (Benner, 1984) and lecturer.

This joint arrangement was the result of time spent in the clinical area, achieving pertinent courses (ENB 124, BSc [Hons] in Advanced Professional Practice) and more recently registering as a student teacher with the English National Board (ENB). However, all these qualifications do not ensure that I can teach or have knowledge, and self-criticism and reflection help me focus on my abilities and learning needs.

I hoped, on being asked to lead the modules, that my clinical skills were appropriate and could be transferred to the classroom setting. I hoped that my clinical background was broad enough to facilitate learning in others, and that my management skills were up to the job of organising and running two modules on a degree programme as well as my current post.

Further, I hoped that my clinical experience would support the application of theory to practice as well as practice to theory. In this situation my expertise should provide credibility in both the classroom and the clinical environment.

Being asked to lead two modules was an honour. It suggested that I was a credible and knowledgeable practitioner who could offer a further dimension to the present degree course. Teaching is something I had wished to pursue for a while, and the opportunity was too good to say 'no thanks'.

However, life is never simple and there are always obstacles to overcome. My role within the hospital was of a clinical team leader and thus I had a number of staff I was directly responsible for. Also, my role within the structure of the cardiac services unit demanded certain roles of me. In order to fulfill the teaching requirements and my present clinical post I needed to negotiate and delegate some of my role.

Operationally my absence during the delivery of two specialist modules resulted in the loss of a staff member for 31 days over a nine-month period. Appropriate remuneration was provided by the university, which allowed for bank staff to fill my absence, but this does not always offer a balanced alternative – it merely offers a short-term stop-gap. Further, the times that I was unavailable for the ward may be at odds with my expected presence at specific operational meetings. Likewise, the ward may require my presence on a day that the university would prefer me to be available for exam board meetings, as an example. Despite such a short-term arrangement, it was still evident that working for two employers has its drawbacks.

Flexibility was the key to this problem. My manager was aware of the commitment placed by the Trust in purchasing places on the degree course and clearly there were expectations on the module, which I was now delivering, to run smoothly. I also had to be flexible in managing the triad of demands on my time, namely, the needs of my clinical environment with the needs of the students, as well as the needs of the university. It is not possible to act alone in these circumstances and communication – informing people well in advance of what is going on, was a key feature in its success.

Being in practice made me more accessible for students than if I had been solely based at the university, as the majority of students were based within the same hospital as I was (there are three hospitals in Leicester). Students knew where I was and could negotiate any further help that they required.

This can have the potential drawback of being inundated with requests for help, as you become too accessible. This has, so far, not been a problem as my students have kept to the arranged tutorial times.

A further advantage of being based in the clinical area was accessing potential speakers for the modules. My expertise lies within a certain scope and I am aware of my limitations outside of these parameters. As one module included aspects of cardio-thoracics, which I have only a little knowledge of, I could identify key people to invite to speak, which resulted in the arrangement of the timetable with moderate ease. If one speaker had to pull out I could potentially invite another at short notice. I arranged both of the modules around the hospital, which also encouraged speakers to attend as they would not have far to come, or have to fit us around their (frequently) hectic schedules.

This local knowledge was useful in arranging rooms for teaching or arranging equipment. The university provided acetates and flip charts, but they are not the only tools for presenting information. For example, one speaker presented their session from PowerPoint, another used an X-ray screen to present X-rays. Having access and availability to these resources was extremely useful and promoted a variety of teaching methods.

Having three hospital sites in Leicester enhanced the variety of experiences for students. Negotiating with the other trusts for time within their clinical areas and inviting key speakers/teachers encourages inter-hospital collaboration, a sharing of resources and benefits the learning of both student and teacher as experiences are shared. This arrangement also facilitates a wider perspective of resources, as students experienced the different management of clinical areas from a more global view. This often curtailed the belief that the grass is not always greener on the other side, nor does one hospital have a monopoly on good ideas or patient care.

Reflecting on the advancement of practice through theory

A major benefit of delivering and leading a module while holding a clinical post is the potential to bridge the gap between practice and theory. A lecturer can provide appropriate, credible information to a class, but may not observe its application in practice. A lecturer-practitioner who works with the same students is in a prime position to explore the theory in practice through facilitating learning in the clinical environment. In order to explore this, the following reflection will be used as an example.

I was working with a student in my clinical area on a typically busy day. The student, whom I shall call Elaine, had been qualified around three years and had worked within the cardiac specialty on another ward. She was familiar with the CCU, but had not worked there before. I knew Elaine fairly well as she had attended one of the modules on which I had taught. We had also worked together earlier in the week, and I was keen to reflect on my facilitation of her learning as a lecturer in practice.

We had established that Elaine preferred to learn from new experiences, where she could link theory to practice. Main (1985) describes this as learning through an activist and pragmatic style which is limited by didactic, instructional methods. Supporting an androgogical approach (Knowles, 1984), the responsibility for learning was firmly placed with Elaine within an environment of safe exploration. This practicum (Murphy and Atkins, 1994) helps the student develop as a professional through safe exploration of dilemmas and their potential outcomes.

Elaine was admitting a patient who had arrived with heart failure and had sought information from me regarding certain aspects of care. As I was interested in the use of theory in practice, I encouraged technical rationality. This use of research-based knowledge (Bines, 1992) was further supported through the use of freedom of a virtual world, where the student can practice in a low risk environment as they are supported by an experienced practitioner. Autonomy is therefore encouraged to support self-learning. This humanistic aspect of learning (Rogers, 1969) is associated with the freedom to make decisions and act on them within the boundaries of defined practice. This situation is reliant on an open and trusting relationship between the facilitator and learner. Concurrently, as Rogers states, when people care for themselves and are cared for by their colleagues, they are then free to care for others (Rogers, 1967).

The androgogical approach (Knowles, 1984) used in this situation supported Elaine in taking responsibility for her own decisions, while linking practice to theory. The development of cognitive skills through androgogy encouraged the use of technical rationality. In discussion Elaine stated: 'I felt my knowledge was good, but wanted some reassurance about a couple of technical things'. In this situation Elaine applied cognitive thought to the observations made, based on previous knowledge and experience. This linking of previous knowledge with theoretical background supports meaningful learning (Mairis, 1992) and was later observed when Elaine applied this knowledge successfully to another patient.

This experiential learning provided the necessary skills for development and the ability to 'bank' the information for future retrieval (Frière, 1972). The complex process of cardiac failure encouraged the need for applying theory to practice. Elaine could later recall this experience as a base to work from with her next patient suffering a similar illness. However, as nursing involves unique experiences, the availability of this knowledge may only be apparent with reflection-on-action (Schön, 1988).

The value of this reflection was consideration of the techniques in use to support learning. The learning environment is influenced by the commitment and motivation of the facilitator (Mairis, 1992) and had Elaine and I not had the time to learn the way we did, I am sure that a more didactic approach may have been used. I was particularly aware that imparting information in an instructional way from 'expert' to 'advanced beginner' (Benner, 1984) may restrict the evaluation of knowledge by Elaine, creating difficulties for me to judge the value of that learning.

This incident was planned and organised with the learner having freedom of a positive practicum to develop in. The facilitation of Elaine's learning was grounded in an awareness and understanding of theory, in this case my understanding of learning theory. If I was unable to consider this I would have been limited in fostering learning within this environment. Concurrently, I feel that Elaine's position would have been untenable without an understanding of theory, in her case the theory of heart failure. By working closely with her, we achieved what we set out to do, link practice and theory where it is needed most – in patient care.

Considering the crumbs

This brief introduction to my role has, I hope, provided some thoughts for teaching in practice. I started by mentioning a cake mix, which I have used as a mental image of the variety of ingredients that influence the facilitation of learning. I strongly believe that practice and theories *of* practice need to be tested through a credible facilitator *in* practice. One way to do this is through the role of lecturer practitioners. However, until there are more of these roles I hope that practitioners consider how and why they learn and teach the way they do.

Key questions and discussion points

❖ What are the advantages of lecturer practitioner appointments?
❖ Conversely what are the disadvantages?
❖ How do staff working alongside people with such appointments view their roles, ie. never 'here' always 'there'?
❖ Does the profession expect too much from these roles?

14.

Novice nurse caring for an expert offender

Sally Rudge

Sally Rudge RMN, RNMH, BA(Hons), Dip Psy, ACBS, MSc is a community nurse working for adults with a learning disability as part of a community based service, which forms a division of a large NHS Trust.

❖ This account describes how a nurse with years of experience may find herself in a novice role despite qualifications and expertise in a range of other areas.

❖ She epitomises the difficult decisions that nurses have to make and the grey areas where simple measurement tools are not available.

My role, as with most community workers, relies upon the assimilation of new referrals into my caseload, active intervention for the caseload itself, and the discharge of clients from the caseload following therapeutic encounter.

The aim of the service is to address the health needs of all adults (19 years+) with a learning disability for the whole county. The community nursing role links with other nursing roles, also based outside of the hospital setting, such as an outreach team, which provides intensive short-term programmes of care, and day centre based nurses who address issues arising specifically at day centres.

The wider links expand through the multi-disciplinary learning disability team, to primary health care teams, voluntary sector staff, and more recently, primary care group initiatives. The community nursing service has an open referral system, allowing anyone to make a referral to the service. All referrals have an initial assessment in which the suitability for the service is decided. If it is deemed a relevant referral, input is planned and implemented. On occasions the referral is found to be more suitable for another discipline, and the appropriate staff are informed.

The majority of my working week is predetermined in terms of therapeutic activity, visiting people with profound sensory impairment, physical disability and mental health difficulties, in their own home, hospital, day centre settings and the independent sector.

My practice has been influenced by a range of theory-based courses in nursing health studies and psychology, however the organisation I work for has adopted a framework based on O'Brien's

(1992) 'Five Accomplishments' for evaluating client satisfaction of community based health service learning disabilities team.

The 'Five Accomplishments' outline five criteria by which a service may be judged in terms of the principle of normalisation and form a framework within which care may be organised. They include:

1. Community Presence.
2. Choice.
3. Respect.
4. Relationships.
5. Competence.

A study by Murray *et al* (1998) found that the 'Five Accomplishments' provided a useful, value based framework for evaluation of customer satisfaction. This was, however, overshadowed by the fact that although the participants were generally satisfied with the service at a therapeutic level, the majority had not been involved in the referral process and had not been given fundamental procedural information. This highlighted rather basic oversights regarding the client's understanding of confidentiality, access to case-notes and information about how to make a complaint.

These are in my opinion a prerequisite to client and carer empowerment, providing the basis for self-advocacy and ensuring professional service providers remain accountable at every level. If the underpinning principle of normalisation is to be achieved, every client needs all relevant information about their care, and the decision about what is revealed to them should not be taken on a 'needs to know basis'.

Wolfensberger (1972) defined normalisation as, 'the utilisation of culturally evaluated means in order to establish and/or maintain personal behaviours, experience and characteristics that are culturally normal or valued.' It is with these concepts in mind that I have shaped both my thinking and practice. This philosophy generates a number of ethical dilemmas, especially with regard to clients who have a sexual interest in children. In these adults the concept of social and cultural constraints and what is culturally and socially acceptable may be beyond their aptitude. Empowerment must operate and be seen to operate within the law, and child protection overrides the personal choice of the client.

There are a number of strategic and operational difficulties that inhibit the development of practice within learning disabilities which primarily relate to the competition of priorities.

My caseload is derived from approximately 700 adults with a

learning disability within my catchment area. To deliver a service to this large geographical spread and disparate client group, requires meticulous planning and a disregard for speed limits. Visits are time limited and to some extent delivered on a rotational system, with some flexibility built in to the working week for urgent matters that cannot wait.

In conjunction with the priorities I set myself, there is an expectation to conform to broader agendas such as those set out in *Health of the Nation* (DoH, 1994), local initiatives and joint agreements with Social Services. Additional issues of equal importance are the need to engage carers and relatives and the development of my own special interests.

These factors could be viewed as an opportunity to develop a professional malaise, burnout or take a ticket on the passive slow boat to retirement. It is my view that these demands create an opportunity to actually achieve job satisfaction, through providing a service which operates at maximum efficiency (one dot on the dial above optimum), and allows me to practice within an arena about which I am passionate.

Some staff believe these inhibiting factors do not allow them to do their job properly and become disillusioned. Perhaps they have not yet recognised that the utopian ideas of health service provision which is free from rationing, are long gone, and we need to do our best with what we have got. I believe that practitioners who perceive a shortfall in service provision should at least make an attempt to understand why their standards cannot be met. I perceive my role as that of a front line rationer, where I find myself rationing services through delay, dilution and termination. This concurs with Klein *et al's* (1996) observations, who suggest that rationing can manifest itself in a variety of ways. It is clear that any financially sound organisation must recognise that resources are finite. However, learning disabilities has always been Cinderella's poorer sister and it is true to say that the provision and apportionment of resources is as overlooked today as it has always been.

The reflective practice cycle

This cycle (see *p. xiv*) should include the following actions:

- start with open questions, eg. 'Tell me in your own words about the pain'
- demonstrate to the patient you are listening, eg. by eye contact, nodding etc
- try to tolerate the discomfort of appropriate silences

- elicit the patient's ideas, concerns and expectations in every consultation
- when satisfied that physical disease is present, always consider its impact on the social and psychological well-being of the patient.

The following scenario focuses on the nursing interactions I had with 'Mark'. It commences with a description of events, followed by a reflection of the feelings engendered in me and concludes with an evaluation of the events. Please note that names have been changed to preserve anonymity.

A referral was made to community learning disability services by a day centre. They were concerned about one of the service users who had recently moved from the family home into an independent flat.

Since moving, his attendance at the day centre had declined. On the occasions he was at the day centre he talked continually about a child who lived next door, and how, now he lived alone he wanted a partner to share his flat.

On visiting Mark, it became apparent that he was staying at home in order to watch Rebecca playing in her back garden. He explained the situation by saying that his childhood and family upbringing had not been pleasant and he wanted to be part of a family in which he saw Rebecca as his sister. Mark's family history involved systematic sexual abuse by his father and uncles, to both Mark and his younger sister. There was no history that Mark had ever sexually abused anyone.

When discussing the behaviour of watching Rebecca, Mark believed he was not doing anything wrong. He said he loved her as a sister, and would never hurt her. He could not accept that others, for example her parents, may not perceive his behaviour as 'normal' or acceptable.

Mark appeared very tense and angry, particularly when talking about his father, and stated that he self-injured at night when he felt at his worst. He described this as thumping and pinching himself and pulling his body hairs out. He found going to bed difficult and consequently was not going to bed until 4.00 am, afraid that his father and uncles may knock at the door. His father and uncles who had been convicted and completed their sentences, lived locally but were not informed of Mark's address.

This incident was important to me in reflective terms, as all my other cases involving sexual abuse have been with known offenders.

Mark presented a conflict of interest – to protect the child, with possible detrimental effects to Mark, or to support Mark and take his rather plausible account at face value.

Feelings

During the appointment I felt confused. Hearing a gentle non-threatening 'caring' man talking about a non-sexual relationship clashed with my (limited) knowledge of sex offenders, their 'typical' cover-up behaviours and the statistics of ex-abused abusers.

A conflicting feeling was that as Mark appeared to have been very close to his sister, supporting each other during the period when they were being abused, he may transfer his feelings for his sister onto Rebecca. If this were the case, Mark would not be a risk to her. However, in overall terms, I felt uncomfortable with his account but was unable to say why specifically.

Following this incident, I felt the need for a multi-disciplinary opinion for the health and social care input for Mark. Mark had invited his mother to the appointment and she was very concerned that his behaviours would 'get people talking' and result in him being victimised. She was convinced that he would not abuse Rebecca in any way. She also stated that Rebecca's parents had spoken with her and were alarmed by the amount of attention Mark gave Rebecca and felt that it was unhealthy – wanting it to stop.

Following the appointment, and with Mark's agreement, a referral was made to social services to reassess Mark's daytime activities.

Referral was also made to psychology and occupational therapy (OT). For psychology, the request was for an assessment of the risk Mark poses to children and for OT to work alongside the community nurse in areas such as anxiety and anger management, together with coping strategies. The OT referral also included an activities of daily living (ADL) assessment which would be beneficial for a social worker with regard to providing appropriate day time activities.

My own role was to continue weekly meetings to assist Mark in coming to terms with his past experiences and to link with other disciplines regarding the recent concerns. Without Mark's knowledge, the child protection unit was contacted to inform them of the unsupported concerns for Rebecca as I felt that Rebecca's needs/rights outweighed those of Mark. This action was taken following discussion and advise from my manager and the Trust's child protection advisor.

Evaluation

All services to whom Mark was referred took an active role. Child protection were confident that Mark was not a current risk to Rebecca, and closed the case. OT work with Mark, encouraging him to practice his newly learned relaxation and anger management techniques. Along with Mark and social services, OT have found more meaningful daytime activities, such as working in a charity shop and dog walking for the elderly. I continue to talk with Mark about his current concerns about his father and uncles. Psychological assessment of risk to others is still ongoing.

Overall Mark's anxieties and anger have reduced and he has good self-esteem. He is 'working' for a large proportion of the week, and has other thoughts and interests apart from Rebecca and having a happy family unit.

Rebecca's parents are more comfortable with Mark and allow contact with Rebecca when they are around.

Mark has divulged information about his abuse to the neighbours and consequently his mother remains concerned that he will be victimised. Although child protection services are not concerned about Mark, I find it difficult to accept their assessment as it was completed without the consultation of other involved professionals. I find myself questioning this assessment, probably as I am still unsure about Mark's behaviours and underlying thoughts about Rebecca.

I have found working with someone who does not have a record of sexual abuse, but who is a potential abuser, very difficult as I do not wish to restrict his quality of life if he is not a threat to others.

Future referrals would probably be more pro-active if they were sent at an earlier stage, ie. at the time of transfer from home to the flat or even before his feelings about the abuse from his father and uncles.

I feel that a community nurses is expected to be a 'jack of all trades', becoming involved in a wide variety of health-related problems. In this case, is there not a potential problem of a novice health care worker 'treating' an expert offender?

Key questions and discussion points

❖ Would you have done the same as Sally in this scenario?

❖ There are many areas of health care where you cannot accurately measure activities or risk. You are left with having to make judgements based on professional experience. What are the implications for this?

❖ The area of sexuality and patient care is difficult and complex. Is this an area where health care practice could be developed?

15.

Lecturer-practitioner: new post, new money, new challenges

Helen Jones

Helen Jones BSc, RGN, Cert Ed FE, RNT, MA works in a large teaching hospital as a senior nurse research and development officer.

❖ This account outlines Helen's strategic involvement in establishing and developing a new and innovative post, something which is often difficult to set up and maintain.
❖ Helen highlights the process of translating an abstract vision into a tangible reality.

New and innovative posts are very difficult not only to set up, but also to maintain. An organisation is unlikely to support a new post unless there is clear evidence that the post will bring benefit and continue to improve the services already available. From inception, they require formal managerial support and detailed planning in order that they are efficient, effective and sustainable. They require organisational structures and processes, some of which will already be in place, in order to maintain them. For lecturer-practitioner posts, preparatory considerations have been published (Jones, 1996a). In my current post as senior nurse research and development it has been possible to realise a personal goal of successfully establishing the post of lecturer practitioner in research.

It is a joint post between The Glenfield Hospital NHS Trust and De Montfort University. The post is currently based in the Department of Continuing Professional Education with both pre- and post-registration education responsibilities. Time is divided equally between the Trust and the university. So, how has this initiative been achieved?

A day in the life of the senior nurse for research and development

I took up this post in 1995. It was one of four innovative posts in a new department. The hospital had recently gained Trust status and only one year earlier had appointed the Director of Operations and

101

Nursing. It was part of her 'vision' to set up the department of clinical practice to support clinical staff in all aspects of their work. The posts would be responsible for education and training, information and manpower, research and development, the fourth post being clerical and administration. The role and purpose of our department demands that we work as a team with a corporate view.

My role as senior nurse research and development means that I have a responsibility for supporting the research and development activities of all the nursing staff in the Trust. With time, these responsibilities have extended to all non-medical staff. Thus the work involves having my own 'vision' which has informed strategic thinking and direction (Jones, 1996b). On taking up post I spent most of the first year working out whom I had a responsibility to work with in the Trust and what I had a responsibility for. Some of the latter was determined by local politics, influencing what I would or would not be 'allowed' to be involved in. I also used this time to begin to establish appropriate networks at all levels within the Trust, across the district, region, and nationally and internationally. In relation to establishing the lecturer-practitioner post in research, networking was essential. Networking is an 'in term' which rolls off the tongue easily in peer group conversations. However, in current times of limited resources – not only in the health care services – it is a real skill that takes time to develop effectively. Working as a true team member also meant that it was necessary to have insight and an in depth appreciation of the work of my colleagues – what was happening in detail in relation to education, training, management issues, personnel and information resourcing. I needed to understand who my colleagues were in contact with and why, and if, and how their work related to my work. Their awareness of my role and responsibilities was equally important. They needed to understand how I was translating my responsibilities into actual support mechanisms for clinical staff in the Trust. For many nurses, the term 'research' is often viewed with apprehension and reserve. I saw it as my role to help de-mystify the subject. In carrying out the post I would be helping to bridge the gap between what is taught and what is carried out in practice. This drove my enthusiasm and provided me with a powerful motivator. It still does today, perhaps even more so now that I have a clearer insight into the barriers and limitations to progress.

Strategic and operational issues for implementing a lecturer-practitioner in research post

There is no doubt that one of the biggest hurdles in implementing a new post is having the appropriate people seriously consider the idea in the first place. It is important to have a proven track record in related issues before you initially expose your 'vision'. In my case, I had already published on the subject and therefore had a detailed appreciation of the associated issues. As my work was quite unique at the time, I was perhaps ahead of many when considering aspects for successful implementation. Holding a senior post in the Trust, I also realised that sound management reasons requiring detailed outcome benefits would be necessary before the post could be considered. As luck would have it, and this too plays a part in any achievement, the region in which Glenfield was a part had for some time taken the lead on supporting lecturer-practitioner initiatives and annual bids were considered. From networking, the partnership with the university was already established. I approached the university, sharing my 'vision' of the lecturer-practitioner in research post and our draft proposal.

It was important to have a document to work from. There were strict criteria for successfully bidding for funding, which meant that the two organisations had to work as a team to achieve the right package. This was good because it meant that both institutions felt ownership of the final proposal. The criteria required the following:

1. The LP would have 50% of their time in service and in education.
2. The bid would provide 60% of total funding of the post.
3. The post-holder, while under part funding from region, must have 20% personal professional development time.
4. The post must be based in pre-registration.
5. The LP post must be a nursing post.

There was no problem with items one to three. The final two criteria caused some concern from the service perspective. While working as a member of the corporate team in the Department of Clinical Practice, it was clear to me that learning was a lifelong experience and that it spanned the pre- and post-registration continuum. Also, in order to have a clinical commitment for 40% of the post (50%, less 10% for professional development) this would have to be with mainly qualified staff. This area of work would provide the outcome benefits of this particular lecturer-practitioner's post. In many ways this, to me, was a major reason for the establishment of the post – to be able to support the application of theory to practice and to be able to demonstrate that the understanding starts in pre-registration and the practical application continues throughout your professional (post-registration) career.

On the issue of the post being just for nursing, again, from a corporate team perspective all disciplines need to work together. In developing a research appreciation and being able to apply it to practice, the worries and limitations of all non-medical disciplines were broadly similar. It would be inappropriate to consider the post uni-disiciplinary.

In confronting these two issues, it was clear that the clinical practice element could be with post-registration.

In discussion with the university, it was also possible to ensure the continuum was maintained in education, although the post-holder would, initially, be based in the pre-registration department. On the concern of being a multi-disciplinary post, it was not possible to find any acceptable alternative other than for clinical contact to ensure that wherever possible, multi-disciplinary research initiatives would be supported. A joint proposal was prepared. The trust and University were required to commit just 20% each of the total costs. Our most difficult hurdle was tracking where the appropriate paperwork had come in to the Trust, outlining the requirements of the bids. However, networking and department team working ensured that we did not miss the closing date for submissions. A week of evening telephone calls between myself and the university, followed by 'next-day-faxing' ensured the submission met the deadline with the correct details and appropriate signatures of support. The first bid was successful in receiving regional support funds and the post commenced in January 1997.

Reflective focus

The first lecturer-practitioner in research took up post on 6 January, 1997. As the person who had initiated this new post it was essential to me to ensure that the findings of my previous study were put into practice (Jones, 1996a). This in itself would then become a living model of theory-practice application. Access and time to attend the local LP forum provided formal peer support. Formal management support was obtained by holding regular meetings with the LP and both the service and education manager. The purpose of the meeting was so that all three stakeholders would contribute and make decisions concerning the role and its undertaking. Any problems could be addressed as a team and realistic solutions considered. Ownership of the initiative would be sustained, which could only serve to improve efficiency and effectiveness. It was intended that a steering group of the initiative would also be established whereby an external advisor would join the LP and the two managers. The external advisor was a research manager from one of the other acute Trusts, who held an unbiased view towards the initiative and could ensure that the focus and direction of the work was being properly maintained. In reality, the four of us worked so well together that we disbanded the managers' meeting in favour of regular steering group meetings. Working well together meant that we each came to the meeting addressing items of concern or success with a critical eye. Meeting the clearly defined purpose and objectives of the post were our prime concern. A formal evaluation was established on an annual basis. Providing evidence of clinical outcome measures for the practice element over a one-year evaluation is not easy. It has been possible to identify indicators of success. Subjective evaluation embraced all aspects of service and education, including tutor and clinical peers and student comments. Individual teaching sessions were also evaluated.

The overall end of year report included an evaluation, which was detailed and informative, and a further year of support funding was offered. On several occasions, I was asked why I felt the post had been implemented so successfully. My response was simply that I had put the findings of my study into clinical practice.

Some six months later personal circumstances left the lecturer-practitioner in research post vacant. While all parties were disappointed at the time, on reflection it actually allowed evolution of the post and changes to the role to be made. We were able to base the post in post-registration, in the Department of Continuing Professional Education. This does include a pre-registration education commitment. It was also possible to offer the post as a secondment opportunity. Also, this time the post-holder is someone who has just commenced a tutor-training course. Having a new person in post has helped once again to take the evaluation one stage further.

In the current climate of radical change and health care opportunities, this post seems to sit very well. Current evidence from the UKCC and the ENB suggest that more and more theory-practice-linked posts are the way forward in the immediate future.

In a world of heavy competition for limited resources, it is inevitable that only those posts that are proven to be effective and efficient in their purpose are supported and maintained. Thus it is incumbent upon the post-holder to provide that evidence from an objective perspective.

The future

The post remains, at present, developmental. In time, it would be more effective in outcome terms if it were not. Conversely, it is a very powerful developmental post for either a clinical nurse to develop their teaching and educational skills or for an educationalist to be supported in the re-utilisation of their clinical skills.

One question is, where should future funding for the maintenance of this post be drawn? It may be possible to make the service contribution from portfolio (research) funding. It may also be possible for the costs to be shared between all the hospital specialities as they all benefit from the support. It is important to acknowledge that the future of the post will be dependent upon a clear identified need for the post. It will have a limited life. But then new alternative roles will be required.

In my view this post will continue after its third and final year of support funding is complete. We hope to take the post across all three acute hospitals in Leicestershire. We also anticipate that the post will become multi-disciplinary.

Key questions and discussion points

❖ Helen talks about her own vision her manager's and the university's – what part does vision play in practice development?

❖ Do you need a proven track record before you risk exposing your own vision?

❖ It took Helen a year to establish this new and exciting post. What are the difficulties in securing long-term funding for posts which do not immediately provide measurable outcomes?

16.

The case for clinical supervision: providing support for specialist practitioners in general practice

Chris Hale

Chris Hale RGN, PN Cert, Moorlands Cert, ITEC has an advisory and facilitative role for nurses working within general practice settings. The account was written as a reflection of her part-time return to clinical practice.

❖ Chris uses a highly structured approach to problem-solving her apparent unease when returning to practice, outlining her involvement with clinical supervision.

I returned to clinical practice following, four years as facilitator for the health authority. My theoretical knowledge had remained updated by providing induction and mentorship for new practice nurses as well as teaching and assessing clinical courses. My post consisted of one day per week at specialist level in a small inner city practice with a second nurse covering a further three days. The basis for this account stems from a telephone call with the 'leaving nurse' following my induction, which had consisted of working alongside her for six weeks.

The nurse stated that she was happy with my clinical skills. I however expressed concern that it was difficult to ensure that practice remained safe and accountable in such an isolated situation, and that the lack of any ongoing support mechanism highlighted this sense of vulnerability. She suggested that I was being unduly anxious but discussion ensued, the outcomes of which were that I would always ask the GP if unsure, continue to read and update and obtain a contact number for the other covering nurse.

Following this communication, I reflected that these measures were not the key to allaying my anxiety, but some continued contact with another colleague was required to discuss everyday work stresses as well as ongoing patient care. I remembered that the other covering nurse had recently undertaken clinical supervision training and contacted her to suggest that we meet on a regular basis for this purpose. She agreed, identifying with the same sense of isolation as I felt.

My initial concerns over the lack of any support mechanism were emphasised by the telephone call which left me feeling upset. However, the empathy of the other covering nurse allayed fears by the realisation that despite years of practice experience she too felt the need for support.

I chose to use Stephenson's model for reflective practice as cited in Palmer *et al* (1994). This poses a list of questions for practitioners to ask themselves after an event, which guide the reflective process:

Q. What was my role in this situation?

I attended my first clinical supervision session having considered some issues which I wanted to discuss. I tried to talk openly and honestly about my concerns and listen carefully to a peer's impression of my views and her feedback and perceptions.

Q. Did I feel comfortable or uncomfortable? Why?

I was uncomfortable at first, feeling nervous, unsure of how the session would go and slightly threatened that this nurse would negatively criticise my practice. I found it difficult to admit that I found my work stressful at times. This was soon to be replaced with a sense of being supported and encouraged.

Q. What actions did I take?

I started with a stilted description of my opinions on the need for peer contact to encourage reflection and continued updating, but in the positive environment I soon started talking openly and ended up taking notes, deciding that keeping a record of the sessions would be useful. A variety of clinical issues were discussed.

Q. How did I and others act?

We were both a little uneasy at the beginning but we had made a cup of tea and soon relaxed, the conversation full of mutual experiences. We had to keep referring to my prepared list to focus ourselves and keep a close eye on the clock to ensure that we kept to our allocated time for the session.

Q. Was it appropriate? How could I have improved the situation for myself, my mentor?

Yes, our actions and reactions were entirely appropriate for the situation. If I had met the nurse before the first session for an informal chat we may not have been so uncomfortable at the start. Otherwise, the situation went well with no improvement required.

Q. What can I change in the future?

I will not get so stressed about my clinical practice and always ensure I find clinical supervision wherever I am working to provide a safe, supportive environment to discuss concerns.

Q. Do I feel as if I have learned anything new about myself?

Identifying the need for support in the isolated situation in which I found myself has proved to me that I am acting as a safe, accountable and reflective practitioner. It has shown that I do constantly ask questions and seek effective solutions within my practice ensuring it remains updated.

Q. Did I expect anything different to happen? What and why?

I did not realise that clinical supervision would be such a relaxed, empathetic and positive experience. I had expected it to be a more formal, critical experience along the lines of teacher/student assessment relationship, perhaps due to its title of 'supervision' rather than the more appropriate 'support'.

Q. Has it changed my way of thinking in any way?

Yes, I now feel much more confident about discussing clinical practice issues, without feeling my status as a specialist practitioner is threatened. We all have different knowledge and levels of experience to share and doing so encourages us to reflect effectively and maintain the best possible care for the patient.

Q. What support is presently available?

No system of formal support is presently available for experienced practitioners. In the year 2000 the UKCC's return to practice programme after a five-year break (UKCC, 1995) will become a statutory requirement but its recommendations for preceptorship (a four-month period of support by an experienced practitioner) only apply to the newly qualified (UKCC, 1993). The system of mentorship generally refers to support for students on placement (Fowler, 1998) and only applies when a course is being undertaken. No guidelines are offered to those commencing a new post and employers induction programmes vary widely.

Q. Why is support required?

Although personally identified learning outcomes were achieved in full by a comprehensive induction incorporating a period of working with an experienced nurse, when looking at the difficulties of remaining accountable for practice according to the *Code of Conduct* (UKCC, 1992), a gap in support was identified.

Q. What is the value of reflection?

Despite reflection in action (Schön, 1983) identifying some continuing help via the telephone call, further reflection on action (Schön, 1983) was required to achieve a solution to the problem. Twinn *et al* (1996) argue that community health care nurses must respond to continued change by constantly adapting and developing practice in order to offer high quality care. This requires practitioners to undertake reflection as identified by Gastrell and Edwards (1996) who also state that the reflective practice approach is similar to that of research and may not be undertaken due to lack of time. However Damant *et al* (1994) agree that in order to maintain professional development, knowledge base and experience alone may be insufficient and that reflection on incidents and comparison of outcomes should be undertaken with a colleague. The value of critical thinking and reflection for practice nurses is also emphasised by Luft and Smith (1994) who suggest that the very nature of the role incorporates making many rapid and varied new relationships, a skill which benefits from regular reflection.

Palmer *et al* (1994) identify that this process can be profoundly difficult, suggesting that it may lead to conflict and personal distress if guidance and support are not available, and state that structures must exist to enable reflection to take place.

The leaving nurse's omission to mention clinical supervision as an option supports the theory that nurses working in relative professional isolation often find it difficult to remain updated (Fowler, 1998), particularly when addressing the issues of development, responsibility for practice and safety of care as defined in *A Vision for the Future* (DoH, 1993). *Nurses Count: A National Census of Practice Nurses* undertaken in 1992 (Atkin *et al,* 1993) discovered that nearly 10% of practice nurses work entirely alone. Although the other 90% do have one or more colleagues within the practice, they are invariably on opposite shifts and rarely meet to discuss care given. It was also identified that nearly one third of respondents had taken a break from nursing before becoming a practice nurse. Of these 67% were not required to undertake the UKCC's return to practice programme having taken a break of less than five years. This demonstrates that even when this programme becomes a statutory requirement, many practice nurses may be returning to a role that can be stressful and isolated (Gastrell and Edwards, 1996) with a requirement to update and maintain their knowledge and skills under PREP (UKCC, 1995) but without a system in place, statutory or otherwise, to support them.

If learning is only supported by the staff within a small practice, it is difficult to judge whether clinical competence is being maintained (Carruthers, 1995). This problem is compounded by the continuous, often major changes within health and social services and more specifically the shift of care towards primary health, which is placing extra stress on clinical professionals working in this area (Twinn *et al*, 1996).

Q. How can clinical supervision meet this need for support?
Clinical supervision has been defined as,

A formal arrangement that enables nurses, midwives and health visitors to discuss their work regularly with another experienced professional. It involves reflecting upon practice in order to learn from experience and improve competence.

Kohner, 1994

Gastrell and Edwards (1996) go as far as suggesting that it may provide the framework required on which to build all of the continued professional education and training needs of community health care nurses.

It has certainly proved to be an effective learning and development tool, which can be used to promote and maintain a high standard of patient care (RCN, 1998). Butterworth and Faugier, also cited in Gastrell and Edwards (1996), state that clinical supervision is an essential requirement where care is based on relationships (as it is in practice nursing) rather than on proficiency in technical procedures.

First mentioned in *New World, New Opportunities* (DoH, 1993) clinical supervision was described as a means of ensuring accountability and providing support, and its implementation was subsequently recommended in *A Vision for the*

Future (DoH, 1993). The UKCC's position statement (UKCC, 1996) emphasises the need for widespread implementation of supervision systems, recommending that all practitioners should have access, but does not make it a statutory requirement.

In direct contrast, Farrington (1996) argues that it should indeed be made statutory. Clinical supervision can be implemented using a variety of methods and models developed by researchers such as Houston, Butterworth and Faugier and Proctor, all cited in Fowler (1998). In the second event Houston's system of 'one-to-one same discipline' was used, which has been identified as the least threatening and safest environment for practice nurses (Fowler 1998). The fear of criticism can also be understood. As Lowry (1998) emphasised, the hierarchical culture within which nurses work can often make requests for help feel like admissions of inadequacy. The appropriateness of the title 'supervision' is questioned by Teasdale (1998), who states that the very word 'carries overtones of restriction and control' and shares the view of the author that the title 'supervision' is misleading. Clinical 'support' has been suggested as a more user-friendly option.

Researchers have also looked at various potential outcomes and benefits of clinical supervision. Important factors include the need for support in two key areas; to reduce stress, and to ensure practice remains up-to-date by enabling effective reflection. Marrow *et al* (1997) showed that clinical supervision encouraged support and thus reduced stress and developed active communication and questioning skills, which enabled reflective and innovative practice. Lowry (1998) cites Bumard, who surmised that clinical supervision provides an environment in which nurses can separate themselves from patients and thus discuss issues with a more detached, objective view.

Positive support has also been shown to reduce the emotional exhaustion frequently experienced by nurses (Firth *et al*, 1986). This same study also identified empathy as important to this helping process, which was highlighted in both the events as positive and useful. Daloz as cited in Palmer *et al* (1994) outlines six skills for offering support:

- listening
- expressing positive expectations
- providing structure
- serving as an advocate

◆ sharing ourselves   ◆ making it special

All of these were identified within my experience of clinical supervision undertaken .

The final stage of Gibb's reflective cycle is the creation of an action plan. In this case no further action was required except for continued supervision and reflective practice. However, thoughts return to other nurses in the same situation. The author would not have been aware of clinical supervision as an option if wider reading had not been undertaken as part of a health authority role and as a result of close contacts with the local nurse education establishments. Action should be taken to raise awareness of the benefits of clinical supervision and to ensure that training, time and resources are made available wherever nurses identify the need.

Conclusion

I chose to use two different reflective frameworks and through clinical supervision also discussed the need for reflection as an essential part of maintaining professional development. After induction is completed, gaps can be identified in ongoing support mechanisms for all nurses, but in particular those working in professional isolation at specialist level. It has been shown that despite no formal systems being available, support is required to undertake reflection and reduce stress. Here the gap was identified at an early stage, enabling a solution to be found through clinical supervision. With Proctor's defined functions of support, education and quality assurance, clinical supervision 'can provide that vital support mechanism for nurses in the demanding environment of a busy general practice' (Fowler, 1998).

Key questions and discussion points

❖ Would you have chosen to analyse your needs in such a structured fashion? What are the benefits of this kind of approach?

❖ Chris demonstrates that she overcame the fear of clinical supervision. Is that fear preventing you from engaging properly in the clinical supervision process?

❖ What other mechanisms could Chris have used to solve the problem?

17.

Unlocking the key worker role

Frazer Underwood

Frazer Underwood RGN, Dip HE Nursing, at the time of writing worked as a key worker on an acute stroke unit.

❖ This account identifies a process of uniting and integrating the work of a variety of professional disciplines to achieve cohesive care packages for a specific client group.

❖ Frazer uses the concept of knowing and 'unknowing' as part of his reflective development. *'A denial of "unknowing" and satisfaction with one's own level of performance may be the most potent block to the development of expert practice'* (Bishop and Scudder,1990).

The Leicester Royal Infirmary NHS Trust (LRI) underwent a radical review and restructuring of patient services between 1994 to 1996. The impact of the changes for nurses and on the organisation of the business process re-engineering project has been well documented from an organisational viewpoint (Morris-Thompson, 1999). This personal reflection of a nurse working in one of the medical directorate's processes, documents for the first time the development of the key worker role.

The neurology process introduced the role of key workers to its two ward areas in 1996, and this was seen as a natural transition that followed the restructuring of the other roles within the nursing team. The process had witnessed the support worker role develop to work more closely with and start to develop the basic skills of the therapy teams. Additionally, the development of the clinical team leader role from the previous ward manager role to one with enhanced responsibilities and duties for the whole of the clinical team brought changes. For these new key worker posts to develop the traditional role of the 'F' grade nurse was challenged. The new posts evolved to meet the clinical nursing expertise required by a quality driven, patient-focused service, and one that embraced a belief in team-based working. The posts were all advertised and six key workers were duly recruited in acute neurology, CVA, and rehabilitation services

The posts were new and had been carefully thought out. They had clear and concise job descriptions, but how these were to be transferred into practice was not clear. There was no role model, as no one had been there before. The model for care delivery fell between primary nursing and case management. The concept is that the key worker forms a team, primarily with the consultant, but also is recognised by the rest of the multi-professional team as the 'key' person to identify with, to deliver the ultimate aim of improving communication and the planning of patient care. Within the key workers job description, the role summary reads: 'accountable for the clinical care of a designated group of patients from admission to discharge within the neurology process'. A major component of the role is to improve the quality and maintain the highest standards of patient care, through the promotion of evidence-based practice and focusing on effective team working within the Trust and beyond. As the roles were new and innovative, freedom was given to all post holders to develop the roles creatively and unhindered.

I had joined the process a month before the posts were advertised and was successful in gaining the post of acute stroke unit (ASU) key worker. I had been working as a volunteer abroad for the previous two years and was looking for a post that offered me an opportunity to creatively develop a role for myself and an identity for a new unit. I had returned knowing that my previous year's experiences in the UK and abroad, focusing on service development and training initiatives, and my commitment to the delivery of good nursing care should not and would not be wasted.

On beginning the post, my typical day started by washing or bathing a patient with one of the support workers following handover. The physiotherapist and occupational therapist arrived on the ward shortly after and took referrals for new admissions, and updates on the known patients' conditions as well as information about outstanding investigations which may encroach on planned therapy sessions. The ASU has only six beds; the medical team reviewed the patients daily, with ward rounds lasting between half an hour to an hour, and all changes to medical care were documented in the nursing care plans. This structured start was short-lived because of the varying demands of the therapy team (pharmacist, speech and language therapist, dietician and occasionally the social worker) who all sought information to plan their intervention. The patients needed care and colleagues needed support. This outline of a typical morning reflects the pure clinical domain of the key worker on the commencement of the post. It was soon evident that time out of the clinical area was necessary, but this time had to be balanced – no one these days has the luxury of an extra registered nurse to cover many days out of the clinical work area.

These first few months were difficult while the team adjusted to the new roles which challenged myself and the two other key workers. Ultimately this strengthened our good working relationship. Support for each other was high, we all shared the same hopes and fears as we started to unlock the door and explore our roles.

It would have been very easy to fall into a nine to five shift pattern, only working Monday to Friday, as this fitted into the majority of activity on the ward with the rest of the multi-professional team. However our belief in providing support to the ward team on late shifts and at the weekend was equally as important, especially as our role focused on maintaining high standards of patient care. The establishment of a rolling off-duty, which ensured all consultant ward rounds were attended by the paired key workers worked successfully and allowed a key worker to work one weekend in three and once a week have a double shift to provide support to the late shift staff. This example of collaboration highlights the need for speciality staff to be seen as part of the generic team and enhanced my awareness that my own area of responsibility represented just a small aspect of a larger picture.

Turning the key — unlocking the role

Munhall's (1993) newly identified pattern of knowing, the concept of 'unknowing', is a component of reflection that carries a great deal of common sense and one to which I can relate. Unknowing is the idea that not knowing or not understanding something will keep the nurse alert to, for example, a practical situation and will encourage the exploration of the 'unknown' to gain further insight and knowledge. Heath (1999) cites Bishop and Scudder's point that a denial of unknowing and satisfaction with one's own level of performance may be the most potent block to the development of expert practice (Bishop and Scudder, 1990).

As the ASU environment was new to both myself and the other members of the multi-professional team we started to question practices and identify the many routines involved in the care of the acute stroke patient. Many patients followed similar journeys through the unit, although interventions occurred at varying times during their stay. Together with nursing colleagues I implemented new documentation which followed a more logical structure, following a new patient's stay and collecting and communicating information in a clear and simple format. Again, the whole process of the patient's journey included other professionals as well as nurses, who deliver care, investigations and treatments to the patient. The notion of care pathways were very new to the team, but supported by the process manager and the consultant, I took forward the mapping of our routine interventions with the patient and co-ordinated the development of our acute stroke care pathway.

The impact of the care pathway saw the nursing role within the unit change considerably. The nurse was empowered to pro-actively manage each patient's stay. As collaborative documentation was simultaneously introduced with the care pathway, the nurse, on the daily ward round was able to represent and give feedback from the other professionals involved in the patient's care to the medical team. Decisions concerning medical management were now able to be made much quicker than had previously been the case.

For example, the nurse would ensure a CT scan was requested on the first day of admission. The prompt for the doctor to request the investigation had been highlighted as essential for effective stroke care management within the unit. The next day if the scan had not been carried out, the request was chased up and an approximate time for the scan discussed with the radiographer. To complete the process, on confirmation of ischaemic stroke by scan, the registered nurse could give the first dose of oral or rectal aspirin against a group protocol which was written to allow best evidence-based practice to be initiated quickly and effectively. Aspirin given to patients with ischaemic strokes will benefit a statistically significant number to reduce death and long-term disability (Cousell and Sandercock, 1998). This demonstrates the nurses pro-active stance in the improvement of care for the stroke patient. Before this, the patient would be at the mercy of the internal mail system, the radiographer's in-patient's box, and the doctor, to look at a scan and to write aspirin up on the prescription sheet.

Through the acceptance of 'unknowing' at the start of this project and seeing what developed from it, learning together as a team and finding solutions to the problems we encountered, the whole stroke team was brought together to focus on the patient's journey through acute stroke care.

Opening up the doors

Echoing the sentiments above, a patient's journey does not start when they arrive on the ward, nor does it finish when they leave. This is a belief that is hard to hold when working in a busy, stressful ward environment, but one I have found important not to forget.

Communication with admission areas like accident and emergency (A&E) or the medical admissions unit needed to be built upon and developed. As the unit can accept direct admissions, it is regularly caught in the middle of things when these emergency admissions areas are screaming out for beds. Pressure to move people out from these areas can result in accepting unsuitable patients. Opening the doors of the unit to patients who have potentially suffered a stroke we have often found 'stroke' to be far from the diagnostic truth, and this does nothing to develop confidence and build trust in our colleagues.

To raise the profile of the unit in these areas and inform staff of its function in assisting acute admissions to the hospital, which should be seen as 'on par' with the coronary care unit, we looked into developing a link nurse for each area. This idea never got off the ground. Looking back or reflecting-on-action as Schön (1983) describes, it is clearer to understand the reasons for failure. So, although interested in stroke, the potential link nurses were too remote from the unit – physically as well as from its ambition and drive for excellence. It is an interesting notion to explore, that the idea of forcing the 'unknown' onto someone else, when they themselves have not recognised a learning need, could lead to failure.

A solution to the problem of the unit's profile in these areas came about more naturally, one that developed through reflection-in-action (Schön, 1983) as we came up against the barriers that halted the development of the link nurse concept.

The ASU had two research nurses attached to it, and as part of their job they carried out acute intervention clinical trial work, and spent time in A&E screening suitable patients. These nurses had the enthusiasm for promoting good stroke care and to raise the profile of the ASU. We therefore enhanced their roles greater in A&E as communicators advocating the benefits and role of the stroke unit. Similarly, the Trust's stroke support nurse linked into the medical assessment unit to provide a patient screening service as well as promoting the unit. This also allowed for the expansion of the support nurse's role to cover the whole of the medical directorate. It allowed her to provide information and advice to all stroke survivors throughout their hospital stay and interface with the community to provide ongoing input to ensure maximum well being for the patient and their family.

Equally, as our relationship with the admission areas was important to get right, it was also essential to look after the back door, to improve communications and develop trust with areas to where we planned to discharge our patients. These areas were either the medical directorate wards or the rehabilitation ward area within our own process. As the average patient stayed only seven days on the unit, for many the majority of their hospital stay was not therefore with us. The belief that all stroke patients are 'heavy' is difficult to shake off and continues to frustrate me. There is a balance with everything, as the unit has only six beds and an average of 350 admissions a year, there will be a need for flexibility to allow it to function effectively. Our discharge criteria are strict and patients leave, in the majority of cases, for the wards to provide a 'care taking' service. For a patient to be moved from the unit there has to be two things in place. Firstly, a discharge plan identifying an ultimate destination for rehabilitation or supportive care and secondly, the patient needs to be receiving their full nutritional requirements either independently, with or without supplements, or via a percutanious endoscopic gastrostomy (PEG).

Development to allow the nurse greater control in actively managing discharge, rather than being a passive participant, allows us to focus on two final areas of practice enhancements which empower the nurse to achieve the unit's discharge criteria quickly and efficiently for each individual patient.

I spent many months collaborating with the District Bed Bureau to address problems during our now regular winter bed pressures within the acute Trusts. The Bed Bureau is the main controller of slow stream rehabilitation community hospital based beds and was an area that was encapsulated and slowed down by traditional beliefs, trying to function in the activity driven National Health Service of the 1990s.

This change in working practice allowed the nurse to part-complete referral forms for slow stream rehabilitation beds, and to fax the referral directly to the Bed Bureau for their immediate action. Before this project the process could take up to seven days. Now, a faxed back confirmation is filed in the patient's notes within a day, and that patient can be transferred from the unit with the accepting ward knowing that they are on the waiting list to their ultimate discharge destination for slow stream rehabilitation.

The key worker role focused on the acute stroke in-patient stay but the wider issues for stroke became very important as the role developed. The care pathway work had provided a solution to improved in-patient management and care and helped other nurses, who worked equally hard, to keep the unit functioning effectively, providing excellence in care and stroke management.

As the door opened to the role, time spent clinically reduced. As I finished the post eighteen months later I spent a day and a half a week on service and practice development work. During my time in the key worker post I was allowed the creative freedom to develop a unique role.

The idea of looking at the whole journey of the stroke patient, beyond the acute unit led to the development of a new post within the trust, stroke services co-ordinator. A post which has responsibility for; providing experienced clinical input into the acute stroke unit and rehabilitation ward (two shifts a week), for supporting and developing the stroke research team, providing staff development and training opportunities within the neurology process and across the Trust, and to facilitate continuous improvements in stroke service delivery – a post that opens the doors to which all staff have a key.

Key questions and discussion points

- ❖ Practice development cannot rely on one innovative person, they must let go of their ideas and allow others to hold the key to quality care.
- ❖ Simple things such as fax back facilities may improve the quality of care and the speed with which the care is delivered far in excess of their initial cost.
- ❖ Creative freedom is needed to develop roles, innovation only develops where it has space to grow.

18.

The role of a clinical team leader and the challenges of paediatrics

Sandra Kemp RGN, RSCN is a clinical team leader in respiratory paediatrics in the Children's Hospital at the Leicester Royal Infirmary.

❖ Sandra describes the role of a clinical team leader and how she has combined management and a clinical role together.

The clinical team leader has a complex and diverse role which spans the responsibility for all respiratory patients, both out-patients and in-patients. I work alongside all the paediatric consultants, some of whom specialise in children's respiratory problems, and with the process manager for children's nursing. Together we have developed the service for the child and family from referral, assessment, and diagnosis to treatment, review, discharge, and liaison with the community, other health care providers and support agencies to ensure continuity of care. The role also involves the development of clinical nursing expertise and standards within the Children's Hospital. I also liaise with the other clinical team leaders within the children's directorate.

Other hospital responsibilities within this post are acting as the 'bleep holder' – covering emergencies and general support to other wards within the Children's Hospital. Also included in the wider hospital role is that of acting as a health and safety co-ordinator, risk management assessor and fire deputy for the hospital.

A typical day

07.30–08.00: This commences with a handover from the night staff to day staff and allocation of co-ordinator role followed by allocation of patients.

08.00: Co-ordination and allocation of nursing care for the shift followed by a check that staffing is satisfactory throughout the Children's Hospital.

08.30: Attend medical handover to establish which wards have had admissions of children with respiratory conditions and to identify which wards have seriously ill children or potential problems.

09.00–14.00: This span of time usually involves direct patient care, either hands on or working alongside a member of staff. This is an opportunity to supervise, advise and do assessments of staff. It allows an opportunity to talk with relatives in a relatively relaxed way and also to teach children, families and staff.

14.00–17.00: This time is normally allocated to any of the following; meetings, individual performance, appraisal and development reviews, off duty, sickness monitoring, human resource issues, clerical, project work, team meetings, interviewing and appointing staff, training, or hospital wide issues. Needless to say, there are many non-typical days which are spent doing other things such as; teaching on statutory study days, attending study days, advising others on specialised care.

I have always seen the role as challenging and having the potential to develop in many different ways. My hopes and fears when I first took on the role were very much combined. I hoped that I would have the confidence and strength to actually take on such a new and complex role and achieve success. However I also had the fear of failing to cope with the demands and not achieving the high standards of individualised family centred care that I strive for.

Team-based working strategy

The idea of 'coaching' evolved as a result of part of a re-engineering process which aimed to put the patient at the centre of the health care service. An initial two-year project was established to implement team-based working focusing on the process involved in caring for the child and family. The aim was to transfer coaching skills to team leaders and process managers. Coaching involved facilitating appropriate training sessions and team meetings. Team leaders were seen weekly to assess team progress, for development of skills learnt from the training sessions and to identify future training needs. The team coach also worked clinically with some teams to help implement effective team working. After six months working relationships, mutual support, clinical skill development and strength as a team were good indicators that coaching was a success in the emergency process, part of which is the respiratory team. Unfortunately, soon after this period individual team training was stopped, due to lack of funding and an increased workload. This resulted in some teams not having the opportunity to build upon skills learnt in the initial training sessions, reducing their ability to address current issues as a team or reflect on performance as a team.

The Children's Hospital was divided into three teams, each with a process manager. These consisted of the elective process; the emergency process and the neonatal process. The elective process is comprised of general surgery; ear, nose and throat, burns, orthopaedics and trauma, dermatology, plastics, oncology, day care and out-patients. The emergency process is comprised of the admissions unit, general medicine, respiratory, neurology and intensive care. The neonatal process is comprised of the neonatal unit.

Each process had a process manager and a process director. Coaching helped to co-ordinate and share ideas and procedures across the three separate processes, creating where possible a single team approach.

Unfortunately there was a period without a process director, followed by a period without the three process managers, and this appeared to have a knock-on effect as people began 'covering' for other roles as well as their own.

Needless to say, although this has caused some practical difficulties everyone worked very hard to create stability and overcome some of the difficulties.

Recruitment is always a topical issue and it is recognised that there is a national shortage of children's nurses. Although a child's stay in hospital appears to be getting shorter, children seem to be sicker when they are admitted and need a higher and more complex level of care. The dependency of children is shown to be higher and therefore staffing levels and skill mix is changing. The opening of a designated children's intensive care unit within the Trust and the setting up of a retrieval service, has had considerable impact on the work of the children's hospital. Every ward has felt the impact and in particular the respiratory unit. It was apparent the previous winter that the intensive care unit found it difficult to cope with the demand for beds and so some of the beds on the respiratory unit were used for high dependency care to supplement the critical care beds. Staffing levels were increased to cope with the demands and staff were given extra training to care for critically ill children.

Reflecting on the last two years as clinical team leader allows me to enjoy what we have achieved, how things have changed and identify plans for the future.

What have we achieved? The respiratory team has worked together to achieve high standards of specialist care for the child and their family. The team has grown together and developed, with the help of coaching, to be motivated and enthusiastic. They are competent team members, working alongside the medical and allied staff to create a happy, successful atmosphere in which to deliver care.

The specialist respiratory nurses have moved their offices onto the ward to become an integral part of the respiratory team. I feel that I have developed my leadership skills over this period in time and that there is a mutual respect between the respiratory team and myself. I was also fortunate to obtain a Trust award, which enabled me to respond to a request from a hospital in Ethiopia. I was able to visit and advise on patient care, ward management and nurse training. Without the support of my team I would not have been able to take up such a challenge, which has continued to be part of my life.

Over this time the team has developed into an efficient group and strength is drawn from individuals in many different ways. Confidence has grown and effectiveness and efficiency go hand in hand. Patient care has undoubtedly improved due to these factors.

How have things changed? Team work has improved throughout the hospital and as a clinical team leader I feel that I belong to many teams, eg. the respiratory team, the ward team, the emergency process team. The management structure has changed, with the role of the clinical team leader emphasising the clinical aspect of the role.

This ensures that the skills of the senior nurses are not lost into management but stay at ward level and directly affect patient care. Patient care has improved because highly skilled nurses stay at ward level and are able to teach and train staff in valuable practical skills.

What about the future? I plan to continue as a clinical team leader but to ensure that the role is periodically reviewed. I intend to keep my clinical skills updated to ensure that I can set standards for others to follow and to act as a role model for future clinical team leaders. I intend to continue my link with Ethiopia by acting as project leader and to facilitate opportunities for others to take skills to the hospital in order to benefit patients and staff. This may involve a considerable amount of my time being spent on both travel and work on the project, but I am committed to professional development of nurses as well as improving standards of care for patients so feel that it is worthwhile.

Reflection

On reflection it has been recognised that the original goal of an 80:20 split for clinical/management time of the clinical team leader was unrealistic. The expectation of this split has created many problems both for the team leaders themselves as well as for support staff. There is no clear definition of 'clinical', although after discussion there is an obvious meaning such as hands on care, medication, tracheostomy care and drug assessments; as well as a more subtle meaning of working alongside staff as a role model and educator and standard setting and supervision.

Each team leader works in a different way and there appears to be no right or wrong way. It is very much an individual approach. Since appointment I have had support from my peer group and management but, most importantly, I have had support from the respiratory team who have allowed me to develop them as well as myself in order to be the success that we are. In an ideal world I would like more staff to be able to create a paediatric respiratory centre of excellence, which would have both generic and specialist nurses who give high standards of holistic family-centred care. As regards my project in Ethiopia, I would like to think that with the help of others I could improve standards of care for the children and offer professional development for the staff – nursing and medical.

Key questions and discussion points
❖ Is the traditional role of the ward sister/charge nurse still relevant in a contemporary health care system?
❖ Should a clinical specialist always be involved in hands on care?
❖ How can we ensure that experienced clinical staff do not lose patient contact?

19.

Developing the capacity to reflect in dynamic psychotherapy

Jim Bailey

From a nursing background Jim Bailey SRN, RMN, BSc (Hons) Psychol, RNT, Cert Ed (FE), Cert Dynamic Psy, Registered UKCP undertook further training as a dynamic psychotherapist and is now employed as a principal psychotherapist within the NHS.

❖ In this chapter Jim examines the importance and role of reflection within his work as a dynamic psychotherapist.

Reflection is a central part of dynamic psychotherapy for both patient and therapist. The ideas presented in this paper relate specifically to dynamic psychotherapy. Dynamic psychotherapy is based upon psychoanalytic theory and practice. It is a process of looking inwards to scan and review one's experience. The word reflection suggests an inquiring but considered frame of mind; a quiet, thoughtful frame of mind.

For the psychotherapist, reflection is the middle phase of a recurring cycle in therapy. First, there is listening to the patient along with experiencing their presence in therapy. Next, follows reflection on what has been seen, felt and said. Finally, comes commentary and interpretation. However, these phases are more conceptual than actual. In practice, therapy is rarely clear-cut. Mostly, it feels like a tangle with these three phases merged into one confusing blend. Reflection is useful when trying to sort out this confusing blend.

For the therapist, psychotherapeutic reflection requires a particular mindset which takes many years to develop. It is a mindset one rarely develops fully and may be likened to a peculiar form of mental suppleness. Each therapist has his/her own personal struggle to develop and maintain a reflective mindset and this means the task of therapy is approached from a personal standpoint.

I will describe three lessons which have helped shape my reflective mindset and therefore illustrate something of my stand-point in relation to psychotherapy. First, however, I will set the scene by outlining the role of reflection in psychotherapy.

Reflection in psychotherapy

Generally, patients seek psychotherapy because of difficulties which arise out of a confusion between the past, which has been problematic, and the present. Essentially, these confusions involve a mix-up between childhood history and current living. (Joan is a fictional character and I have altered aspects of my clinical illustrations to ensure patient anonymity.).

Joan keeps choosing partners that mistreat her just like her father mistreated her mother. The roles and behaviours both parents adopted in their marriage have been imprinted in Joan and at crucial times they appear in her life. Sometimes she acts like mother, sometimes like father and sometimes like both. Past and present are confused. The confusion is often subtle, complex and unconscious; Joan can be totally unaware that sometimes she acts like her parents did.

When a patient walks through the therapist's door he/she brings these unconscious historical confusions into the room. The task of therapy is to throw some light on these confusions and reflection is a primary tool for this purpose. Typically, patients use therapy to reflect upon their childhood history and current life. This is an intimate, sometimes painful process that starts to bring alive the patient's historical confusion in therapy. The conditions of therapy (ie. the room, the allocated time, the quiet atmosphere) coupled with the therapist's listening stance bring patient and therapist closer together. In fact, at an unconscious level, they become mixed up together. The patient projects into the therapist and more generally the whole therapeutic situation, figures and features from their early life. They are then drawn to relate to therapy and the therapist accordingly. This is the process of transference. Transference and counter-transference are key concepts in psychoanalysis and dynamic psychotherapy. They are primarily unconscious elements of the therapeutic relationship. The evolution of these complex concepts has lead to a situation in which these terms have different layers of meaning and may be used differently. In this chapter, I use the terms in the following ways: transference occurs when the patient transfers, in thought, something from their inner world (often relating to early life) into therapy and the therapist. The impact upon the therapist and what they feel as a result of the transference, is referred to as counter-transference. When these projections connect with the therapist and they identify with the patient's early figures, this process is called counter-transference. Transference and counter-transference are corresponding processes that lead to the therapist getting inside the patient's historical confusion. I wish to stress that these are unconscious processes that cannot be engineered – they happen. Also, they are a necessary feature of therapy and their avoidance, which may also occur unconsciously, will rob therapy of a vital source of therapeutic energy.

Reflection has a significant role to play in unravelling the processes of transference and counter-transference. Particularly, the therapist needs to recognise the patient's transference projections and how they have responded to them. Sandler (1976) describes this deep level of interaction in terms of a need for the therapist to be 'role-responsive' to the patient. For example, cancellations by patient or therapist, are often key points in therapy. They can have an emotional charge because some aspects of the patient's historical confusion is activated. If we consider Joan again: a break in therapy may well leave her feeling neglected (like mother) while her therapist might feel unconcerned and pleased to have a respite from Joan (like father). This is a transference/counter-transference replay of an earlier situation in Joan's life. If the therapist can catch sight of this situation through reflection, then it may be possible to interpret the roles played out.

This form of therapeutic work has the potential for making therapy feel more alive and relevant for the patient. Also, the therapist will feel more tuned in to the patient. However, it is not easy seeing and reflecting on these moments in therapy. It is a difficult task which may be likened to catching a ball. If you snatch at the ball/moment it eludes you. It is much better to wait for the ball/moment to come to you. This requires patience. For the psycho-therapist, patience is a therapeutic virtue.

This catching analogy is apt but because human interaction is so complex, the therapist requires a reflective mindset with a capacity to catch more than one ball at once. A feature of psychotherapy is that several things may be happening on different psychic levels all at the same time. One Christmas, a friend gave me a present of three brightly coloured juggling balls and a ludicrously brief set of instructions. A fascinating thing about juggling is that in theory, almost anyone should be able to juggle because it involves basic hand eye co-ordination skills. Of course few people can, because juggling is, quite simply, unnatural. The skill involves utilising natural abilities to do something unnatural and this is also the case in psychotherapy, where the natural skills used are relating, communicating and thinking. With Joan, at one moment her mother may be evident, at another her father and somewhere Joan is there herself. The therapist's reflective mindset needs to be able to see and catch hold of all these figures revealed by the patient. The only way to learn to juggle is to practise. The only way to learn to be a psychotherapist is to practise.

Not thinking, not knowing and uncertainty

Before thinking, one should have something to think about. This statement may seem to express the obvious, but premature thinking from the therapist can be a major interference to the patient's therapy. Nature abhors a vacuum and the desire to fill a thought-less space is strong. Learning not to think is a deep and difficult skill. The danger of premature thinking is that the therapist may end up reflecting on something that has come more from their own mind than the patient's. At these moments the patient ceases to be the primary focus of attention. At the most basic skill level, the therapist must be able to wait patiently until the patient provides something, verbal or non-verbal, to be thought about. At a deeper level of skill, the therapist must learn to quieten the mind and achieve a state of calm receptiveness. Bion (1962) described this state of mind as reverie and likened it to a mother's receptiveness to her child. In her reverie mother receives the baby's terror and anxiety, brought about through hunger and pain, and then she thinks of how to soothe her baby. However, as any mother and any psychotherapist will tell you, sometimes you do not know what causes the baby's/patient's distress.

The desire to 'know' like the desire to 'think' can exert a distorting pressure in the therapy and Casement (1985) offers the following quote from John Keats (1817) as a guideline to therapists.

> *Negative Capability, that is, when a man is capable of being in uncertainties, mysteries, doubts, without any irritable reaching after fact and reason.*

The therapist who has 'negative capability' leaves the stage clear for the patient's story to be told and for its meaning to emerge in due time. Inevitably, this means the therapist will experience a good deal of not knowing and this is accompanied by uncertainty. Uncertainty is difficult to bear and the desire to resolve it is very strong. This desire can distort our reflections. Patients also hate uncertainty and may well entice their therapist into premature thinking and knowing.

Invariably the knowledge arising from these collusions is of little value because the wish is not for true self-knowledge, the wish is to be rid of uncertainty.

'She loves me... she loves me not' is a child's game where petals are picked from a flower one by one in order to magically know if your sweetheart really loves you. This is a game about not knowing and the desire for certainty. You only know if you are loved when the last petal is removed but this need to know destroys the flower. The lesson of this child's game is that the need for certainty can be destructive.

Doubt is a particular form of uncertainty and extremely common in therapy. The whole process is doubt-ridden for therapy is a world of bits and pieces, hints, changes of mind, conflicts and mere glimpses of truth. Doubt is an uncomfortable aversive state and self-doubt particularly so. However, it is worth remembering that doubt and self-doubt exist because there are at least two possibilities to be borne in mind. Sound therapeutic reflection requires being able to see both options even though the discomfort caused by doubt makes thinking difficult. Self-doubt is rarely far from the therapist's mind and this can be especially uncomfortable for uncertainty is focused upon oneself. I believe, however, that self-doubt is a realistic and therefore a healthy state of mind for the therapist. The desire to quickly resolve self-doubt can lead in two directions. Negatively, it leads to a guilty self-admonishing frame of mind, 'I'm useless and no good at this job'. Positively, it can lead to a state of grandiose denial, 'I know I'm right because I've got a talent for this work'. Both are false resolutions to self-doubt and draw one away from the difficult task of reflecting upon the true quality of one's therapeutic work. Also, these false solutions can distract us from reflecting on the patient's historical confusion and how we may be enacting a part in it. In order to bear self-doubt the therapist needs a core of healthy belief in him/herself and in psychotherapy as a treatment. This core belief provides the foundation for sound and secure practice. Put simply, one has to believe in oneself and in what one is doing.

The desire to think, know and resolve uncertainty or doubt can all have negative effects on the patient's therapy. Learning how to manage these 'desires' is an important step in developing the correct mindset for therapeutic reflection.

Survival first

Freud (1912) recommended that therapists approach their work in a particular frame of mind. They should be in a state of readiness but without specific expectations of the patient. He coined the term 'evenly suspended attention' to describe this frame of mind. He also made a corresponding recommendation to patients. He said they should 'free associate'. This meant they were required to say whatever they thought. In psychotherapy today there is a tendency to encourage communication or allow patients to discover the value of openly expressing their thoughts rather than giving instructions to free associate. However, the principle of Freud's idea remains valid. His recommendations to patient and therapist outlined the conditions under which psychotherapeutic reflection could take place. The open and clear minded therapist combined with the freely communicating patient create the ideal therapeutic couple. This ideal situation is rarer than one might hope for. Frequently, therapists are faced with great frustrations and challenges to their 'evenly suspended attention'. The therapist's capacity to think can be severely tested and attacked.

To illustrate how one's thinking may come under great pressure I will briefly return to juggling. There are some performers who juggle using chain saws. This daring feat must involve great skill coupled with a mastery of fear. By contrast, many patients seeking psycho-therapy have suffered fear during childhood that could not be mastered because they were children and the fear was too great. This fear may be lodged inside them in an unconscious unprocessed form. When this un-mastered fear emerges in therapy it can sometimes be deposited into the therapist because it is unbearable. At these moments survival may be an issue at the centre of the patient's historical confusion. I recall a patient who frequently faced me with the frightening task of catching a vicious 'chain saw' part of her personality. This part of her would be kicked into life if, to her way of thinking, I got something wrong. She had a considerable intellect and coupled with her vicious streak I became easy prey. I would rarely predict her chain saw assaults when, after sweeping into my room, she would proceed to condemn me as useless and I would feel cut down. During and after these episodes I found it extremely difficult to reflect. My capacity to think was shredded and all I could do was try to find a place somewhere in my mind to hide. This was how I survived these chain saw attacks and it took me a long while before I was able to think and reflect upon them. This patient had in fact been subjected to random chain saw attacks on her psyche by a disturbed mother. This mother could suddenly switch from being sickly sweet to vicious and taunting. Her attacks came out of the blue.

In therapy I became mixed-up in this patient's frightening historical confusion. I was made to experience some of her childhood fear and this paralysed my capacity to think rather like she had felt bewildered as a child. Undoubtedly, this patient was psychically scarred and in turn I suffered some scarring at her hands. However, I learnt more from this patient about survival and thinking while in fear than many of my less demanding cases. I have found that difficult patients can teach one more about being a therapist, but the lessons they offer are usually hard ones to learn.

Limitations

One of the first patients treated through psychotherapy described her treatment as 'the talking cure'. Although this term has become slightly modified over time to 'the talking treatment', it captures some key essence of psychotherapeutic work. Words, talk and language are at the heart of psychotherapy. However, patients struggle to find words to describe their experience, past and present. And likewise, therapists struggle for words to make sense of what they hear, see and feel in therapy. For the therapist, this language struggle is twofold. First, it involves finding a personal reflective language. There is no reflection without language for even if one thinks visually, it is language alone which makes sense of the visual image. Second, the therapist must find a language that is accessible to the patient, one that enables them to communicate. This second factor involves the complex area of therapeutic interventions and rather than stray into this realm of technique, I will continue to focus upon reflection.

Therapeutic reflection is structured and limited by the language we possess. It is the primary tool for our reflective thinking but in truth it is a feeble tool. Language is like a spoon and the task is to empty a bath full of water using nothing else. Sometimes we tilt the spoon or turn it upside down and we carry no water, we find no meaning. Frequently we fail and all the while the task is greater than the tool we possess. Each session contains more material than can be gathered up and made sense of and therefore each session presents the therapist with more than they can cope with. This is particularly noticeable when patients bring a number of complex dreams and present them all in one session. The sheer quantity of the material can feel overwhelming. The possibility of being overwhelmed is always lurking in the wings and can take centre stage at any time. This is an inherent part of psychotherapy and because of this strange situation, therapists are faced with their inevitable limitations. This, of course, is fertile ground for self-doubt but it is most important to become familiar with the limitations of one's reflective capability, for this realism reduces the risk of elevating oneself or psychotherapy onto an unrealistic plane.

There is also something else to be learnt from the situation described. The limitations inherent in therapy reflect something of the human condition. They show that life cannot be mastered and controlled and because of this they reveal how weak and vulnerable human beings are. Many patients seek psychotherapy because they cannot bear the weak vulnerable aspects of themselves. They may develop false solutions which temporarily hide their weaknesses, but false solutions have their costs and eventually drive people to seek help. Often there are very good reasons why patients feel weak and vulnerable. For example, a Jewish man once told me in an omnipotent fashion that if he had been in a concentration camp during the war, he would have had the strength to survive. I was shocked and this set me thinking of the holocaust – the massive horrendous scale of it, the systematic brutality and how pervasive it was. I also thought of how weak and vulnerable one would feel inside a concentration camp. This was too much for me to comprehend. There was a limit to my reflective capability. I did recognise, however, that my patient was also at a personal limit. He could not bear to face something about the horror of his own past and how weak and vulnerable it left him. He shocked this inability into me and I recognised this from my inner reaction and the omnipotent way he talked about the concentration camp. Significantly, this piece of material arose as we began to concentrate upon how weak and vulnerable he could feel, but sadly he left therapy abruptly. My lesson was to appreciate my patient and I both had limits to our reflective powers.

The lessons I have outlined are probably common ones for most psychotherapists. However, they are lessons that can never fully be learnt for they recur in different guises with different patients. Through these lessons there is a continual testing of one's capacity to reflect. This constitutes a pull towards development in the therapist which, I suspect, mirrors a pull towards development in the patient. Without the ongoing trial of these lessons something would be missing from psychotherapy.

Key questions and discussion points

❖ To 'develop his practice' Jim undertook further training and is now employed as a dynamic psychotherapist rather than a nurse. What are the advantages and disadvantages of this model of practice development?

❖ Many nurses give serious consideration to re-training in some other form of the helping or therapeutic profession. Is this because suitable opportunities and developments within the nursing profession are simply not available?

20.

Reflection on a role in practice development

Rachel North

Rachel North RGN, RHV, DPSN, BA (Hons) is a directorate nurse advisor and has a role to facilitate professional development within a large community trust.

> ❖ Rachel's role involves encouraging practice development initiatives within a community setting. She reflects on how the role has developed over a number of years.

Prior to taking up this post I had trained as a general nurse and worked as a staff nurse for a number of years, principally in oncology. I then trained as a health visitor and practised as a family health visitor before moving into research related to sudden infant death syndrome. I worked as a research associate for four years and during that time also gained experience in training, policy development, service evaluation and lecturing.

When I was first appointed to my current post it was on a fixed term contract to cover the maternity leave of the existing post-holder. I was used to being employed on short-term contracts and, since I had little specific previous experience of a professional development role, I preferred to have the opportunity to 'test the water' without being committed to a longer-term contract. Initially, the range and diversity of the work that was involved overwhelmed me. It consisted of a large number of distinct projects ranging from developing records for different service areas to developing and implementing policies to support practice. In each case it required me to work with other practitioners and managers to agree what needed to happen and how. To draft and re-draft the necessary documents and supporting papers for agreement by the Trust Board and dissemination throughout the organisation, and then to support implementation of change in practice.

Each day would involve:

- Responding to requests for information from practitioners and managers either about work in progress or for advice on how to respond to a new problem or initiative that was impacting on their work.

- Meeting to discuss different projects with the relevant working groups and agree the next steps towards formulating a policy, developing tools to support good practice or implementing change in practice.

- Gathering and synthesising relevant evidence both within and outside these meetings to ensure that the various projects were soundly based.

- Drafting documents ranging from minutes of meetings to policies, clinical guidelines, records and explanatory papers.

- Responding to *ad hoc* requests, for example, to draft a response to the latest Government Green Paper on some aspect of service provision or professional practice.

- Providing training and making presentations to groups of managers and practitioners to support practice developments.

As time went by the enormous challenges of the work became increasingly fascinating and are explored in more detail in subsequent sections of this chapter. Suffice to say, I am now into my fourth year in the post and still learning.

As I became more familiar with the scope of my professional development role a number of things became apparent. First, my role was to work with nurses in the Trust. However, the reality of clinical practice meant that issues affecting nurses often affected other clinical practitioners equally, and implementing change in clinical practice almost always required the involvement of other clinicians. Second, my research background was both helpful and a serious handicap in this role. The nature of the research in which I had been involved was such that I was used to knowing a lot about very little, now I needed to know relatively little about a lot. The focus had shifted from narrow and deep to broad and shallow. This induced in me a constant fear of never knowing enough to feel confident about the judgements I might be making.

Another consequence of my research background was that it had trained me how to think, but in a particular way. I was used to analysing and organising large amounts of complex data, but my reasoning was inductive rather than deductive and had its basis in a rational, scientific model. The data that I was handling now was diverse, often qualitative and requiring pragmatic 'real world' resolutions. I lacked the models 'in my head' to help me to make sense of such data and present it in ways which were applicable to the world in which I now found myself. I found it all too easy to miss whole steps that were critical to successful implementation of often complex practice developments.

I was also very content focused. Understanding a subject in depth, being willing to submit my work to the scrutiny of others and accept that it would undoubtedly be pulled apart mercilessly were all requirements of carrying out research. The important thing after all was the quality of the work. Quality of work content remained an issue in this post, but added to this was the need to consider the quality of the processes used to carry it out. Working with people added a whole new layer of complexity to getting the job done. Added to this was the need to understand the context within which practice development needed to take place. Recognising real constraints on not just what was achievable but also how something could be done within those constraints, was essential to achieving effective approaches to development.

This also meant understanding the different perspectives that different people with different roles could bring to bear on any subject. It was important to recognise the value that these differing perspectives could bring to reaching a satisfactory outcome, rather than seeing blocks and barriers.

Finally, language is a powerful tool. Unfortunately, the language used in academic circles is often very different from that used by practitioners and managers. Initially I found that every time I sent out a memo I would be inundated by 'phone calls from the recipients asking me to explain what I wanted. Learning to present information and ideas in ways that matched those in which people thought in their everyday work, using language that was accessible was evidently an urgent requirement.

The example I have chosen is a simple one but demonstrates all the issues described above. I was asked to contribute to a project that was already under way to explore how the care of housebound diabetics could be improved. This work was building on a survey which had been conducted by two practitioners within their own caseloads who had identified that housebound diabetics were less likely to receive regular reviews of their diabetes than those who attended clinics at their GP practice.

It took two years to develop an assessment tool which could be used by district nurses to assess diabetics in their own homes, and associated training and guidance on agreeing practice protocols to establish systems within GP practices to ensure that housebound diabetics received annual reviews.

The reason it took so long was two-fold. First, I lacked the necessary process skills to explore issues with a multi-disciplinary group and gain a clear picture of what the problems were and what needed to happen to resolve them. Second, I needed to develop a systematic approach to analysing practice development requirements to ascertain their scope. For months I met with practitioners from nursing, dietetics and chiropody and regularly became mired in technical detail about diabetes and operational detail about its management in primary care. They each brought a wealth of knowledge and experience to the work but also different perspectives and ways of thinking through problems. They clearly had the necessary expertise to help me to identify what was needed, but I was unable to ask the right questions. Indeed, much of the time I was too busy trying to find answers to even start asking questions. In the end I was helped partly by their unending patience and partly by some other work with which I was involved, which started to give me some of the knowledge and skills I needed to do my job.

The first step forward came when I read about the Job Competence Model (Mansfield and Mitchell, 1996). This model describes the four types of skills which people require in order to perform effectively at work. These skills are technical, task management, contingency management and managing the work interface. Technical skills are those which are specific to the job you're doing.

Task management skills are those which are involved in prioritising and organising your work. Contingency management skills are complex skills that involve anticipating and responding to different events or breakdowns in systems. Practitioners use contingency management skills every time they work with a client, adapting plans of care to suit their individual requirements. Managing the work interface is another highly complex set of skills relating to how you work within a set of physical, social and organisational constraints and develop effective working relationships with colleagues and clients. This model gave me a conceptual framework within which I could analyse practice development requirements. It was now possible for me to organise the information which my colleagues gave me and to draw coherent conclusions about what was needed to support the care of diabetics in practice.

I also used this model to explore how I was working on this project and it quickly became clear to me that my task management skills needed some attention. Because this was a relatively small project compared with some of the other work in which I was also involved, I realised that I wasn't giving sufficient dedicated time to it between meetings. By setting aside a day to work through all the issues that had been discussed and to process the information available to me, I was able to save potentially hours of 'bitting and bobbing' and never quite getting the work finished.

The second source of help came partly from working with an external consultant whose work involves facilitating individual and organisational effectiveness and partly from the work of EH Schein. Schein (1987) describes a model of working with people known as process consultation. Process consultation is very like the process of clinical supervision. The focus is on helping your 'client' to identify a problem and find ways of resolving it. The critical feature of process consultation is therefore about how you structure your relationship with your 'client'. The relationship is essentially a 'helping' or enabling one, rather than one in which you take on an expert role and provide all the answers. Reading Schein's (1987) work made me realise that, in spite of my complete lack of knowledge and experience of managing diabetes in primary care, I had nevertheless been assuming an expert role within the group. Believing that I had to provide answers I had failed to ask the questions which could help the group to work out the solutions. No wonder it was taking so long and we seemed to be going backwards so much of the time.

This combination of a model, which could help me to ask the right questions, and a more effective process for working with people, significantly improved my ability to make progress with this project. I still found though, that I experienced difficulty in understanding the different ways in which members of the group thought through problems and how they related to each other. Here again I was helped by the literature. In *Really Managing Health Care*, Iles (1997) describes the different ways in which people think, across a range from concrete detail to abstract concept. Each has its place and having as wide a range as possible in a group is now something that I actively seek to achieve.

Doing so invariably improves the quality of the work. It does however require more management. Abstract conceptual thinkers often appear 'airy fairy' and 'not in the real world' to more concrete thinkers. On the other hand, concrete thinkers tend to appear slow and plodding to the conceptual thinker who quickly becomes bored by their attention to detail.

Iles (1997) adds two further dimensions to this analysis, one in relation to how people like to work and the other in terms of what motivates people. Again, understanding these factors and how they influence the way in which a group of people work together allows the development of processes which build on individual strengths and encourage group cohesion.

The next time I met with the group I analysed the individuals' different styles of thinking, working and what seemed to motivate them. I then tried to use that knowledge to channel their contributions to the project in ways that played to their strengths and helped to build the relationships within the group.

When I reflected back over the two years of the project, I became aware that the most significant personal development over that time was in the shift I had made from focusing on the content of the work to concentrating on the processes used to carry it out. There were two strands to this. The first was understanding the different skills that were needed to fulfill a piece of development work, the second was making that understanding work for me. Those skills on which I had to work hardest were my task management skills and those associated with managing group processes and facilitating development.

Learning to set aside sufficient 'thinking' time regardless of all the other competing priorities which we all have to manage in our work is often a real discipline, but one that invariably pays rich dividends in the end. Developing skill in facilitation or process consultation is probably what the concept of lifelong learning is all about! It's become practically second nature now to watch and learn from how others work with individuals and groups, to analyse group processes and to reflect on my own practice and what worked and what didn't in any given situation and identify why that might be.

Recognising that in this kind of work I will always be learning has also encouraged me to consider how I learn best. When I explored this particular example I realised that it's important for me to have a blend of 'hands-on' experience, the opportunity to work with others who have greater expertise and can 'model' ways of working and then the theory starts to make sense and to provide a richer understanding. It is my hope that these insights will help me in future as I continue to refine and develop my skills.

Key questions and discussion points

❖ Should managers drive change or facilitate it?
❖ To what extent is practice development a strategic team approach or an individual's innovative vision?

21.

Reflections in the mind

Dr Deenesh Khoosal

Dr Deenesh Khoosal LLM(RCS), LLM(RCP) (Ire), BAO, MB, BCh, FRC Psych works as consultant psychiatrist, clinical tutor, and also as an examiner for the Royal College of Psychiatrists.

❖ Deenesh considers the process of becoming a psychiatrist and the consequent roles and responsibilities this position holds.
❖ He reflects upon the relationship psychiatrists have with other disciplines, together with the most and least enjoyable aspects of being a psychiatrist.

The concept of reflections on development in practice is invaluable in helping practitioners understand what is done, how to make some sense of everyday practice and to learn by experience. The reflective practice cycle described earlier in this book offers a model for this. The chapter also suggests that this mechanism should allow similar situations to be better handled in future. I fully endorse this. I propose to reflect on the major issues facing psychiatrists today.

How does one become a psychiatrist?

A psychiatrist starts his career by training to become a doctor at medical school. When this training is completed he becomes a qualified medical practitioner. Qualified medical practitioners then specialise in one of several areas that is of interest to them, such as medicine, surgery, psychiatry, etc. If psychiatry is chosen then the medical practitioner spends several years as a trainee in psychiatry itself. This training starts at a senior house officer level and then at the specialist registrar level. The psychiatric trainee will learn about mental health, psychology, mental illness, sociology, statistics, etc. as required by the Royal College of Psychiatrists. The trainee will need to pass the MRCPsych examinations of the Royal College of Psychiatrists to qualify as a psychiatrist.

The psychiatrist then functions as a senior trainee learning the specialist skills necessary to be a consultant psychiatrist. In my case,

I entered Medical School in 1972, qualified as a medical practitioner in 1978, passed the MRCPsych exam in 1983 and became a consultant in 1986.

What does a psychiatrist do?

A psychiatrist is a specialist medical practitioner who is qualified to assess patients who are referred, to reach a diagnosis and to formulate a management plan. There has been much discussion over the years about terminology for those people who consult doctors from clients and service users through to patients. In this chapter I will refer to this group of people as 'patients'.

Assessment and diagnosis

Assessment and diagnosis are usually the chief role of the psychiatrist. A detailed assessment covers the problems a patient is currently experiencing and relates these to past history, personal history and general functioning. As religion, culture, background, etc. also influence how an illness is experienced, these factors also need to be taken into consideration. The assessment, therefore, provides information necessary to reach a diagnosis.

Management

The diagnosis determines a management plan. This plan can consist of physical, social and psychological interventions as appropriate.

Physical measures range from medication appropriate for the illness to electroconvulsive therapy and even psycho-surgery in those rare instances where it is indicated. Social management is necessary for those patients with social difficulties such as assisting with rehousing, benefits, etc. Psychological intervention ranges from supportive psychotherapy to cognitive therapy, individual analytical therapy, and also includes anxiety management.

A competent consultant psychiatrist needs many skills. No single person is ever likely to possess all these skills. Most consultant psychiatrists, therefore, work closely with other professionals who make up the community mental health team. The community mental health team I work with has a psychologist, social worker, community psychiatric nurse and occupational therapist. We are also able to obtain other professional help when necessary, eg. dietician. The combined skills of the multi-disciplinary team are more likely to meet the needs of the patient.

Branches of psychiatry

There are several specialities in psychiatry, for example the psychiatry of learning disability, psychiatry of old age, general adult psychiatry, child and adolescent psychiatry, liaison psychiatry, etc. Psychiatrists working in these specialities have undergone further rigorous training in the chosen branch and usually devote the rest of their professional career to that field. They are often at the forefront of research, service development and service provision in these areas.

Teaching

Most psychiatrists are involved in teaching undergraduates where there is a medical school. Psychiatrists are also involved in postgraduate education, teaching, research and audit. The Royal College of Psychiatrists strongly encourages this and regards consultants doing this work as 'educational supervisors' to their trainees. All consultants need to demonstrate participation in continuing professional development themselves as required by the Department of Health.

Place of work

Most of a psychiatrist's work takes place on an out-patient basis. To gain access to the service, the patient contacts the general practitioner who sees the patient and then makes a referral to a psychiatrist if necessary. A small number of patients need assessment at home or in-patient treatment.

Legal obligations

The Mental Health Act (1983) is a legally binding Act of Parliament which governs the detention of patients who are mentally ill and who need to receive compulsory treatment in hospital. Psychiatrists must adhere to the provisions of the Act. Compulsory detention with treatment is only contemplated where the patient will deteriorate if treatment is not given. Most patients are treated on a voluntary basis.

The difference between a psychiatrist and a psychologist

Some people are confused about the difference between a psychologist and a psychiatrist. A psychologist is a practitioner who obtains a university degree in psychology (usually a BA) who then chooses to specialise in clinical psychology. He will apply for training in clinical psychology. A qualified clinical psychologist is then able to offer psychological interventions though many psychologists choose a sub-speciality such as cognitive therapy, behavioural therapy, etc. Some clinical psychologists obtain a PhD in psychology and are addressed as 'doctor'. As they are not medical doctors, they cannot prescribe or supply medication.

There is a some overlap in the work done by a psychiatrist and a psychologist. Most good psychologists I know choose to work with psychiatrists just as most good psychiatrists I know choose to work with psychologists. Helping the patient to recover with appropriate intervention is the target of both practitioners.

What are the major issues for psychiatrists today?

Like most specialist fields psychiatry is constantly changing. There have been numerous developments that have been responsible for this such as a greater understanding of brain structure, receptor sites, psychopharmacology, working with families, etc. Never has there been a time in the history of psychiatry when so much is happening. Perhaps the prophecy that there will come a day when a vaccination will become available to prevent schizophrenia will come true.

There have been developments from the Department of Health too. The *Health of the Nation* (DoH, 1992) identified specific mental health targets, such as a reduction in the suicide rate. Health Trusts are working hard to achieve these targets at a time when there has been increased reporting of murders committed by psychiatric patients, frightening the rest of the population into thinking that all psychiatric patients kill despite evidence to the contrary. The plethora of statutory enquiries into homicides is indicative of the level of concern.

Personality disorder is another area that has demanded attention. There has been much debate about the best way to provide services for patients who are so personality disordered that they pose serious problems not only to themselves but to others also. The Government has recently issued a document on the management of personality disorders, though the issue of civil liberty and conclusions from Ashworth Prison provide considerable insight into this complex area.

The Mental Health Act (1983) which reflected public thinking at the time is probably out of date now. Further changes to the Mental Health Act are being planned. One area that has been extensively debated is how to compel someone to have treatment in the community. The needs of the patient and the needs of society need to be balanced in this complex matter. As medical practitioners British psychiatrists have resisted being used as instruments of the State as their duty to the patient must remain paramount.

The greater availability of drugs and alcohol has imposed further problems for individuals, their families and their community. These mind-altering substances can dramatically influence not only the onset of psychiatric illness but also its progress. They can also make pre-existing mental illness worse. Psychiatrists argue that patients need to be encouraged to participate in their recovery and to assume responsibility for themselves. This is a far cry from the 'nanny state' where people insist on rights but appear to take no responsibility for themselves or for their recovery.

What is the best part of the job?

Despite all the pressures I personally enjoy my work. Well, most of the time anyway. I enjoy the opportunity of working closely with people. The opportunity of developing a working relationship within which therapeutic goals can be identified, methods to achieve these gains devised, and monitoring progress, seem to me to be an invaluable way to work. Linking up with other professionals in promoting recovery offers considerable pleasure when someone recovers. Most patients know that psychiatrists do not have a magic wand to make problems disappear. Psychiatrists can help patients greatly by involving them in their own recovery. Recovery is tempered with sadness too as recovery is associated with discharge, for remaining involved beyond this time could stand in the way of progress.

What are the disadvantages?

There are some disadvantages for psychiatrists just as there are in any profession. My greatest complaint is about the volume of paperwork that needs to be completed for each patient contact. Unfortunately this is necessary as it forms a record of that contact, not only for further therapeutic work but also for medico-legal purposes. My second dislike is when I have to compulsorily detain patients for treatment purposes. It seems so sad to need to do this at what is usually a frightening and intrusive time at a vulnerable point in someone's life.

My third regret is related to the volume of work. Where I work the ratio of the psychiatrists to the general population is substantially below the prescribed norms of the Royal College of Psychiatrists. This means that I am unable to give as much attention as I would like to some things, such as one to one work with individuals. My fourth regret is the increasing number of complaints that are made by patients or their carers. This suggests either that society is becoming more litigious or that psychiatrists are not meeting the needs of some of their patients: reasons such as being overwhelmed by demands of patients, being bogged down by paperwork, inadequate training, etc. Complaints generate even more paperwork which can make a bad situation worse.

Increased recruitment to medicine and encouraging the retention of trained doctors are two major thrusts employed to ensure that the public's expectation for health provision is met. Recruitment to psychiatry has also been a problem area though measures currently in place are not likely to improve the situation until the medium term.

My final regret is the stigma that accompanies mental illness and for patients who are mentally ill. Clearly this stigma is not as intense as in the past. This is largely due to publicity campaigns by the Royal College of Psychiatrists, increased awareness of mental health matters and greater willingness by patients to seek help from psychiatrists. Unfortunately much work still remains to be done to reduce this stigma.

Future

If I had the choice again I often ask myself would I choose psychiatry as a profession? I believe that the answer to this lies not so much in someone choosing to study medicine as medicine choosing that person. Special skills are needed to become a psychiatrist after this. Despite these drawbacks I would have no doubt about choosing psychiatry as a career option again.

In this chapter I have reflected on my career choice and vocation. I now come full circle to the reflective practice cycle through evaluation of my feelings, conclusions and future plans. While psychiatry will never be all things to all people, there is no doubt on reflection, that psychiatry can help, does help and will continue to help.

Key questions and discussion points for the reader
❖ How can we assist professionals to spend more time giving direct client care and less time in administrative roles?
❖ What further work can be done by practice development staff to reduce the stigma of mental health problems within the wider community?

22.

A short view of professional development

Dean Hart

Dean Hart RMN is a day hospital manager and practice development nurse.

> ❖ Dean gives an honest and very personal account of difficulties that arose early in his career and how those problems were solved.

During the early part of my nursing career I found it very difficult to maintain focus, and I am sure that others will have experienced similar difficulties. I found that pressures of work created a situation where my main objective was simply to go to work to 'do the job' go home and get as far away from it as possible. (I am sure this will not sound unusual to other nurses who find themselves in similar circumstances.)

My own experience is representative of the above. Early on in my career very significant life events had sapped me of my enthusiasm and motivation. It was all I could manage to actually go to work. My personal life has always been my priority and my career a very definite second place. During this period it was nigh on impossible to contemplate my professional development. Being truthful, I did not really know what it meant. My time and energy were spent working through personal problems. I had completely lost sight of my career and was not really concerned. My professional development was stalled and it appeared that my career, such as it was, was stagnant. The frustrating thing was that all of the time I was aware that I had the potential to succeed. However, I found that it was impossible to figure a way out of the mire. People began to notice and became concerned that I was merely functioning. It was only then that I began to realise work was not going away. So what do I do now?

This rather negative view of myself, my career and the prospects on offer, prompted some serious reflection. Subsequently, a number of questions as to how I could develop a positive solution for myself and for my employer who was starting to notice my, let's say, 'relative lack of interest'.

Probably, the easiest answer would have been to ask for help, but that did not occur to me. I found it extremely hard to have the

148

capacity to maintain any kind of self-awareness to extricate myself from this predicament. It actually took my nurse manager to approach me. This was a strange experience as he asked to see me outside of work 'to discus my career'.

Very surprised I agreed, but afterwards thought to myself 'here we go'. I had decided this would be a 'shape up or ship out' discussion. It turned out to be something very different.

Yes, in the ensuing discussion, there was an element of 'shape up or ship out', but the 'meeting' was mainly concerned with the fact that someone had noticed I had potential. This struck me as puzzling as it was incongruous with the feedback that I was receiving from my ward manager. Gradually I began to comprehend that it was about my making choices and seizing my career 'by the scruff of the neck', and my deciding on the way forward. It would be an understatement to say that this had a dramatic effect on me. It became obvious to me that my career was an important part of my life and that it could help improve my self worth at that time.

As my manager stated, 'It is difficult to start to climb the ladder of development when you feel you are at the bottom, but once you start to climb and get up there, motivation to keep up-to-date and enthused and motivated is far easier to maintain.'

All I had needed was someone to point this out to me. This did not mean that the 'road to recovery' was easy after that, but it at least gave me something to latch on to. Gradually, I began to apply the skills I knew I had and my motivation and enthusiasm returned and increased. In the process, colleagues began to appreciate my contribution to the workplace and most importantly to patients. This gave me an immense sense of professional well-being. Over time I began to think about where I wanted to be along the professional continuum, realising that I did not want to stay a staff nurse indefinitely.

However, it is important to realise that even once insight is gained, your professional development is partly still dependent on the quality of educational opportunity and the availability of organisational commitment and sponsorship. You should not do all your development in your own time.

My next step was to wait for the right post to come along. This turned out to be a post as deputy manager of a day hospital for the elderly. Shortly after this (for once being in the right place at the right time), I was promoted to manager. This meant I was now not only responsible for my own development but that of a team of nurses.

It was important for me to consider the experience I had had, before examining the needs of other individuals. This was also a challenge for my own development, which I quickly realised was sometimes dependent upon where your colleagues are along the professional continuum. By that I mean you have to adapt to the needs of each person and the level of guidance they need, and their development can be a reflection of your own. It is about using my experiences positively, creating an environment that allows others to develop professionally.

For my part, my own professional development, like many other forms of development, is an internal process. I found that the key to my professional development was being able to identify my own unique attributes, realise more fully my own capabilities, and utilise them to their optimum effect. It can be easy to become lost in nursing's attempt to attach itself to academia. If you remind yourself of the fundamentals of nursing practice and where your skills fit in along that continuum, then you should be able to adapt, refine and develop your skills accordingly. But it helps if you have a mentor to guide you through the initial stages.

There are four principles I use to guide myself through the varied ideals of professional development. These are not academic principles, but more personal tips that I have found useful:

1. I try to engineer a conducive environment in which I can develop.
2. I try and maintain an awareness of my abilities.
3. I now always find an ally, (someone who can offer you objective insights).
4. My professional development is my responsibility.

The moral of my story is now clear: professional development is your own responsibility, but it helps if you can find an ally that will make the transition to a high degree of commitment, motivation and success a supportive rather than painful experience.

Good luck to anyone who reads this account and benefits, it will then have been worthwhile and thanks Andrew for his insight.

Key questions and discussion points

❖ How typical is Dean's story of phases in your own career?
❖ Would a more structured clinical supervision have helped Dean in the earlier part of his career?
❖ What can we learn about organisational effect on individuals which gives rise to similar problems?

23.

Now I'm free(lance): reflections on me by me – where to now?

Andrew Clark

Andrew Clark RMN, RGN, Cpn Cert, ENB 955, FETC, DMS, MBA currently works clinically in Accident & Emergency and independently as an educator in both private and NHS health care settings.

❖ Andrew reflects upon a complex career with varied roles and an unexpected turn of fate which resulted in a complete change of career direction.

Most people after a long (or short) time become a little fed up with their lot. I am no exception. I have enjoyed a long, varied career (mostly in psychiatry) and for the most part have relished my nursing background and the pursuit of excellence within it with a passion (which has sometimes created animosity amongst less motivated colleagues as well as friends). This is my story very much in précis. I hope that anyone who feels at a loss can use my experience. If this is the case then the effort required to actually commit this to paper will have been worthwhile.

Over the last year I have had the opportunity to reflect in depth on my career as I have spent the best part of the year working in a freelance capacity.

The early part of my career was spent working in psychiatry. My training which started on the 13 September, 1976 was relatively uneventful, although I enjoyed my general nursing secondment and the community allocation to the CPN department (community psychiatric nursing service). From that moment on I wanted to be a CPN.

After a couple of years as a staff nurse in psychiatry I was bored and felt that I was not progressing and, in the absence of any career advice, I decided to undertake my general training. By and large except for the odd spot of unnecessary formality I enjoyed this spell, though personal circumstances dictated that I should return to psychiatry.

Having returned to psychiatry I then tried to pursue my long standing ambition to become a CPN. On the third try I was finally successful gaining a post in the elderly team. It was a liaison advisory post to the ten Part 111 homes in a mixed rural and urban patch in the north of England. The sense of freedom as I left the hospital gates behind in a colleague's car was amazing and I can honestly say that I have never enjoyed going to work so much in my life. Every day was a discovery and the freedom to plan your own work routine and the order of the work was excellent.

After a couple of years working as a CPN my then manager sent me on the ENB 811 (CPN Cert) at the Continuing Nurse Education and Nurse Research Unit based at the Royal Victoria Infirmary in Newcastle. This was my first real experience of an academic based course and although I found the travelling hard work it served to increase the motivation factor. After the course I spent a great deal of time teaching in the training school and felt that that was the way forward for me.

I enjoyed my teaching but despite being asked to apply for a post another candidate was chosen and swallowing my disappointment complete with the lumpy bits, decided to try management as I thought I might enjoy the problem-solving aspect of the role. Thus I was duly appointed as a clinical nurse manager for a community mental health team. The stress factor multiplies here as there are ever constant demands from senior staff to partake in both clinical and management based activity without any real time allowance being given to either. After a short while managing a community based service, I moved to manage the in-patient services for the elderly. Managing ten or so staff is easier in comparison to managing 420 odd. If you think that it is stressful and hard work managing an essentially nine to five service, you should try managing 24-hour services.

Although I relished my operational management post with its (metaphorical) 'fire fighting' and problem-solving role, after five years I needed a change and further challenge being somewhat tired of the constant 1.1% cost improvements required at the time (1.1% of an 8.5 million budget does not seem like much but after four years of cuts I felt that there was nothing left to cut).

I eventually left my management role for three reasons: firstly, due to personal circumstances (no elucidation necessary on these pages at least); secondly, I had become tired of the endless budgetary constraints; and lastly, I was keen to try a more facilitative practice development role. Maybe if the right post arrives I will go back to management but until then there are other challenges which are equally enjoyable.

Recruited to a community practice development role which, for a number of reasons, turned out to be not quite like it should have been. Having ensnared the individuals, promised resources were not available and the service wanted more of a managerial function than my colleagues and I were prepared to feel comfortable with.

The decision about what to do next however was taken for me. After fours years and a short secondment to set up and run a new course, my 'fixed term contract' which by virtue of time had become substantive was terminated and I was redundant. What do I do now was the pressing question. I was well qualified but the roles I had ceased to provide me with the challenges I needed. It was now important to discover something that not only paid the bills but, equally important (perhaps more so), that I enjoyed.

I turned down several quite lucrative managerial offers from the private sector and decided to return to my roots, do some bank work and re-discover what it first was that made me become a nurse.

It would have been too easy to dwell on the negative aspects of that time in my career and the temptation to reveal the depths of particular individual's lack of awareness and stupidity was sorely tempting. In the end though it would achieve little. Negative emotion is seldom fruitful. It is far more appropriate and ultimately useful to have a positive outlook throughout your struggle to re-establish yourself.

The experience has taught me a great deal about human behaviour. Colleagues that one expected to be able to rely on were few and far between. Perhaps it is often the case that those you feel should be helpful often cannot be for whatever reason. However, people you expected to be unhelpful were very supportive. Only a very few colleagues reacted in the manner that I would have expected. Many senior staff who could have helped did not for fear of their own position in the reorganisation process. Very clearly, loyalty (which I treasure) is in short supply, something I found personally very sad.

Any reflection is essentially a personal process and an insight to me may well be obvious to someone else. Analyse you own circumstances before transposing my experiences into your own frame of reference.

Reflecting on my own career has provided me with different insights at each phase.

My move to my general training was my first real step on the development ladder. If you are not on the ladder it is hard to take the first step. Once you are on the ladder and motivated it is far easier to maintain your development. Unfortunately, I got to my 'dream post' rather too late (CPN) and had to move to other things as I needed a role which provided me with further challenges. Management brings rewards in terms of financial rewards and the ability to have a greater influence and help staff develop but equally it has its problems. They can be risky in terms of security, they usually cause stress, grey hair and a dramatic reduction in one's social life as the volume of work can be staggering, with constant pressure to increase output from limited resources. By far the best part of being a manager though, was the ability to be in a position to nurture talented staff and watch them grow professionally into senior practitioners. This is one of the few parts of the role that I still miss to this day.

Practice development has less pressure but in some ways is harder work as you have to compete with the management agenda and competition for funding, either for yourself or others, can be even more intense. Many organisations undervalue continuing education and seem to effectively ignore the ability and effect it can have in motivating staff long-term. Despite the cost it is invariably money well spent.

I have been fortunate that in every job that I have had, somewhere I have encountered fantastically motivated individuals who have helped me along my journey of self-development. I have been and still am constantly amazed at the quality of staff that I encounter on a daily basis. Despite everything that their respective organisations and the political arena can throw at them, they persist with a commitment to quality patient care which is a pleasure to behold.

I am now in the privileged position of operating a portfolio approach to my work. I spend the majority of time in clinical practice (this time in the general field in Accident & Emergency, utilising my psychiatric skills to good effect) and (although temporarily I hope) at the bottom of the money tree. To make up for this I spend some time teaching nursing at a university and some time working in a freelance capacity in psychiatry. I never get bored and my time management skills are better than even when I was a manager.

For those staff who find themselves in the position that I was in, my message is simple. Take your time to re-discover yourself and what you now want from your career. It is too easy to rush into something just to provide security. The professional qualifications you have can earn you a living at whatever and wherever while you decide. It has only taken eighteen months to put together a portfolio which provides a salary which is more than my previous practice development post. I am aware that I am relatively well qualified, though it was my analysis of skill based qualities that led me to make the decision about what I was going to do.

If I can do it so can you

I am now entering a another new phase of my professional development and I have not enjoyed going to work so much for many years. I also do not think that I would like to return to just doing one job. The variety which I now enjoy is so stimulating and brings its own rewards over and above the financial aspect of things.

Whether I return to a more managerial role or even return full-time to psychiatry, I have not yet decided. I need further time to contemplate and cogitate. Doubtless, in the fullness of time, I will come to a decision of sorts which will move me in another direction, whatever that may turn out to be. I am lucky in that I have retained the motivation and drive that some others have lost. To a certain extent I have to thank reflection for assisting me in this complex task.

Reflection will not solve all of nursing's or an individual's problems nor will it provide answers to unasked questions. But to engage in the reflective process in a positive fashion will ensure that you are as equipped as you can be to deal with whatever should come your professional way.

Key questions and discussion points

❖ Would you have dealt with the change in the same positive way?
❖ What other alternatives might Andrew have considered?
❖ How typical is Andrew's story?
❖ For practitioners with diverse interests and qualifications, does the current nursing career structure restrict individual's flexibility of movement?

Reflections on reflection

The notion of reflection is one that many health care professionals learn about in school, perhaps write a two thousand word assignment about, and is considered an admirable and positive quality experience for everyone else, but an experience that we never really get around to doing for ourselves. Critical self-reflection is described by Morgan (1996) as a cornerstone of modern healthcare practice, yet the practice of reflection for most professionals appears to be 'dead in the water'. This is probably due to a range of competing factors which traditionally include, 'lack of time', 'patients come first', 'I don't need to reflect because I'm good at what I do'. I would suggest that although these reasons may have some legitimacy, they invariably exclude the fear of critical analysis of one's own attitude, opinion, prejudice, behaviour and professional performance. This fear stems from the professionalisation of healthcare, that is, the individual cultures which have developed policy and procedure to a level where professionals become extremely apprehensive if they feel their practice will be exposed as falling short of 'gold star quality'. Any deviation could result in professional suicide.

To some extent the development of clinical supervision has provided a safe environment where mistakes can be obviated outside of the managerial or disciplinary process, however clinical supervision may still present a host of risks for the supervisee, not least in terms of confidentiality. Reflective practice on the surface appears to be an excellent solution to the manager who is unwilling to support the development of clinical supervision due to a lack of time and resources, and the practitioner who is fearful of disclosing their thoughts or weaknesses in professional practice. Reflective practice is an activity which requires few resources, as it is invariably undertaken alone and without technological assistance.

The proposition that a development of critical thinking skills requires educational involvement beyond the level of basic preparation, (Schank, 1990) gives rise to the possibility that the main reason for the lack of reflective practice could be that professionals just don't know how to do it. If this is the case, then the ability to reflect is not a natural phenomenon, and must therefore be promoted through education.

Minghella and Benson (1995) proposed that critical incident analysis is a valuable method of promoting reflective nursing practice and as a tool for developing curriculum content, however their espousal only serves to help us fall into the trap of focusing upon the extra ordinary rather than the ordinary.

I was once asked at interview to extol the benefits of reflective practice to an eagle-eyed, elephant-eared interview panel, at which point I froze. Not because I was unable to recall the theory, but because to give real consideration to the subject one needs to be able to feel confident about self-disclosure, and my discomfort with this reflected in my failure to secure the post.

Self-disclosure and reflection are not necessarily synonymous, although an introspective disclosure to oneself is reflection. Oscar Wilde (1894) proposed that 'Only the shallow know themselves', a phrase which hints at the complexity of being human, and perhaps some of the intangible aspects that make up the 'self'.

Reflection can be seen as a continuum that has casual consideration at one end and an exploration of both sub and unconscious material at the other. The textbook definition of what is and what is not reflection constrain the process to the middle of this continuum, and fail to explore the extremities of the spectrum through either self enlightenment through meditation, or the internal acknowledgement that accompanies a minor mistake. Theories also fail to recognise the link between unconscious automatic behaviours, which are changed by events, as in Pavlov's classical conditioning, and the conscious process postulated in Wilkinson's (1996) all-encompassing definition of reflective practice. Here, reflective practice was seen as an active process, whereby the professional can gain understanding of how historical social and cultural, cognitive and personal experiences contribute to professional knowledge acquisition and practice.

Once personal reflection is committed to public scrutiny it is contaminated by the fact that other people may interpret the content. In our legitimate efforts to decipher and seek meaning from another's thoughts, we may attempt to empathise with the substance of the material, but that empathy is the same superficial empathy we hold for a character in a novel. Perhaps our ability to identify with the character in this novel and the consequent emotions which emerge, directly determine how we might rate this book, and consequently, the value we place upon it. Likewise, if we have difficulty in relating to, or empathising with the reflective content written by another, then there is a risk that it will be rejected or dismissed as no good, or of little value by the reader.

However the whole point of reflection has very little to do with the reader, and any insight or benefit the reader may gain is secondary to the objectives of the reflector.

So, assuming there is an inherent danger in committing one's reflections and therefore oneself to paper, the authors of this book have taken a personal risk in sharing their thoughts, feelings, successes and failures to enable you, the reader, to gain insight into their world.

Unlike an autobiography or travel diary, the motivation to donate the very personal accounts is solely driven by the reflector's understanding of the paucity of real reflective accounts in contemporary texts. The contributors to this book were, with one exception, persuaded to relinquish their anonymity in the interests of credibility, however, each one understands the personal and professional risks which committing these reflections to paper incurs. It is with this in mind that the reader might be persuaded to accept the reflections as the true thoughts and feelings of the contributor, and use these as the basis for generating discussion with colleagues, or posing questions for the reader's own practice.

The range of events, experiences and insights this book unveils is testimony to the complex and diverse world of contemporary health care, in which each individual practitioner interfaces with circumstances that build into an experience base over time.

Considering the idea that reflection and particularly professional reflection, should be a journey which is somehow transformative for the traveller/reflector, it is surprising that it is eschewed by the majority of 'learned and informed' workers. Eco (1987) suggested that the ubiquitous urge of almost every child to visit the hyper-reality of Disneyland is the very same drive that motivates a Christian to embark on a pilgrimage to Lourdes or Rome.

This symbolic road to personal and professional enlightenment is captured by the process of reflective practice. If only Bilbo Baggins or Dorothy from the Wizard of Oz had known about reflection, they could have reduced their journey time, and saved a great deal of effort.

References

Abram SE, Reynolds AC, Chancellor MB (1983) A comparison of analgesic effects of electroacupuncture, placebo acupuncture and transcutaneous electrical stimulation. *Anaesthesiol Rev* **10**(10): 26–31

Adam S, Osborne S (1999) *Critical Care Nursing Science and Practice.* Oxford University Press, New York

Andrews M (1996) Using reflection to develop clinical expertise. *Br J Nurs* **15**(8): 508–513

Andrews M, Gidman J, Humphreys A (1998) A reflective practice. Reflection: does it enhance professional practice? *Br J Nurs* **7**(7): 413–4, 416–7

Argyris C, Schön D (1974) *Theory into Practice: Increasing Professional Effectiveness.* Josses Bass, San Francisco

Atkin K, Lung N, Parker G, I-Erst M (1993) *Nurses Count: A National Census of Practice Nurses.* Social Policy Research Unit, York

Atkins S, Murphy K (1993) Reflection: a review of the literature. *J Adv Nurs* **18**: 1188–92

Benner P (1984) *From Novice to Expert: Excellence and Power in Clinical Nursing Practice.* Addison Wesley, California.

Benner P (1988) *From Novice to Expert: Excellence and Power in Clinical Nursing Practice.* 2nd edn. Addison Wesley, California.

Bines H (1992) Issues in course design. In: Bines H, Watson D (eds) (1992) *Developing Professional Education.* Society for Research into Higher Education and Open University Press, Buckingham

Bion, WR (1962) A theory of thinking. *Int J Psychoanalysis* **34**: 306–10

Bishop A, Scudder J (1990) *The Practical, Moral and Personal Sense of Nursing.* State University Press of New York, Albany, New York

Boud D *et al* (eds) (1985) *Reflection: Turning Experience into Learning.* Kogan Page, London

Boyd E, Fales A (1983) Reflecting learning: key to learning from experience. *J Humanistic Psychol* **23**: 99–117

Brodie Welch LB (1979) Planned change in nursing, the theory. *Nurs Clin North Am* **14**: 307–321

Burnard P (1995) Nurse educators' perceptions of reflection and reflective practice: a report of a descriptive study. *J Adv Nurs* **21**: 1167–74

Butterworth T, Faugier J (1992) *Clinical Supervision and Mentorship in Nursing.* Chapman and Hall, London

Campbell A, Edgar S (1993) Teenage screening in a general practice setting. *Health Visitor* **66**(10): 365–6

Carruthers P (1995) Support and supervision. *Prac Nurs* **3**(II): 379–82

Carver J (1998)The perceptions of registered nurses on role expansion. *Intensive Crit Care Nurs* **14**(2): 82–90

Casement P (1985) *On Learning from the Patient.* Tavistock, London and New York

Cheng RSS, Pomeranz B (1987) Electrotherapy of chronic musculoskeletal pain: comparison of electroacupuncture and acupuncture-like transcutaneous electrical nerve stimulation. *The Clinical Journal of Pain* **2**: 143–149

Cousell C, Sandercock P (1998) *Antiplatelet Therapy Compared To Control In Acute Presumed ischaemic Stroke.* The Cochrane Library

Damant M, Martin C, Openshaw S (1994) *Practice Nursing Stability and Change.* Mosby, London

Darbyshire P (1993) In the hall of mirrors. *Nurs Times* **89**(49): 26–8

Department of Health (1989) *Working for Patients, The Health Service. Caring for the 1990s.* HMSO, London

Department of Health (1991) *The Patient's Charter.* HMSO, London

Department of Health (1992) *The Health of the Nation, A Strategy For Health In England.* HMSO, London

Department of Health (1993) *A Vision for the Future, Nursing, Midwifery and Health Visiting Contribution to Health Care.* HMSO, London

Department of Health (1993) *Changing Childbirth: Part 1 Report Of The Expert Maternity Group.* HMSO, London

Department of Health (1995) *Supervised discharge: The Patients in the Community Act.* HMSO, London

Department of Health (1993) *Mental Health Act, 1993.* HMSO, London

Department of Health (1994) *Health of Nation Key Area Mental Health Handbook – Seeking Local Views Supporting Advocacy Services.* 2nd edn. HMSO, London

Dewey J (1933) *How We Think.* DC Heath, Boston

Dickens C (1986) *Martin Chuzzelwit.* Penguin Classics, London

Donovan CF, McCarthy S (1988) Is there a place for adolescent screening in general practice? *Health Trends* **20**: 64

Eco U (1987) *Travels in Hyper–reality.* Picador, London

Edwards SD (1996) *Nursing Ethics. A Principle Based Approach.* Macmillan Press, London

English National Board (1991) *Framework for Continuing Education.* ENB, London

References

Farrington A (1996) Clinical supervision: UKCC must be more proactive. *Br J Nurs* **5**(12): 716

Firth WB, McIntee J, McKeown P (1986) Interpersonal support amongst nurses at work. *J Adv Nurs* **11**(2): 273

Flint C (1990) Taking the reins. *Health Service Journal* June **28**: 969

Fowler J (ed) (1998) *The Handbook of Clinical Supervision – Your Questions Answered.* Quay Books, Mark Allen Publishing Ltd, Wiltshire

Fraser RC, McKinley RK, Mulholland H (1994a) Consultation competence in general practice: establishing the face validity of prioritised criteria in the Leicester Assessment Package. *Br J Gen Pract* **44**: 109–13

Fraser RC, McKinley RK, Mulholland H (1994b) Consultation competence in general practice: testing the reliability of the Leicester Assessment Package. *Br J Gen Pract* **44**: 193–6

Freehan J (1996) *Evaluation Of A Teenage Screening Programme* (Unpublished)

Frière P (1972) *Pedagogy for the Oppressed.* Penguin, Harmondsworth

Freud S (1912) Recommendations to physicians practising psycho-analysis. In: *The Complete Psychological Works of Sigmund Freud.* Vol 12, 111–20. Hogarth Press, London

Gastrell P, Edwards J (eds) (1996) *Community Health Nursing Frameworks for Practice.* Baillière Tindall, London

General Medical Council (1993) *Tomorrow's Doctors. Recommendations on Undergraduate Medical Education.* GMC, London

Gibbs G (1988) Learning by doing: A guide to teaching and learning methods. In: Palmer A Burns, S Bulmer C (1994) *Reflective Practice in Nursing: The Growth of the Professional Practitioner.* Oxford Scientific, Oxford

Gordon J (1982) Acute complications. In: Guthrie DW, Guthrie GW (eds) (1982) *Nursing Management of Diabetes Mellitus.* 2nd edn. Mosby, St Louis

Hall DMB (ed) (1989) *Health for all Children, A Programme for Child Health Surveillance.* Oxford University Press, Oxford

Hall DMB (ed) (1991) *Health for all Children, A Programme for Child Health Surveillance.* 2nd edn. Oxford University Press, Oxford

Hall DMB (ed) (1996) *Health for all Children, A Programme for Child Health Surveillance.* 3rd edn. Oxford University Press, Oxford

Harbermas J (1971) *Theory and Practice.* Heinemann, London

Hargreaves J (1997) Using patients: exploring the ethical dimension of reflective practice in nurse education. *J Adv Nurs* **25**: 223–8

Hastings A, Fraser RC, McKinley RK (in press) *Student perceptions of a new integrated course in clinical methods for medical undergraduates*

Heath H (1999) Reflection and patterns of knowing in nursing. *J Adv Nurs* **27**: 1054–9

Hibble A, Elwood J (1992) Health promotion for young people. *The Practitioner* **236**(Dec): 1140–3

Hullat I (1995) A sad reflection. *Nurs Standard* **9**(20): 22–23

Hunt C, McDonnell A, Millan C (1996) *Becoming a Reflective Practitioner*. University of Sheffield Press, Sheffield

Iles V (1997) *Really Managing Health Care*. Open University Press, Buckingham

James CR, Clark BA (1994) Reflective practice in nursing: issues and implications for nurse education. *New Educ Today* **14**: 28–40

Jarvis P (1992) Reflective practice and nursing. *Nurse Educ Today* **12**: 174–81

Johnson G, Reynard K (1994) Assessment of an objective structured clinical examination (OSCE) for undergraduate students in accident and emergency medicine. *J Accid Emerg Med* **11**(4): 223–6

Jones HM (1996a) Introducing a lecturer-practitioner: the management perspective. *J Nurs Manage* **4**: 337–45

Jones HM (1996b) *The Research and Development Strategy for Nursing 1996–1999*. The Glenfield Hospital NHS Trust, Kandaprint, Leicester

Jones E, Williams C (1993) Growing awareness. *Nurs Times* **89**(49): 29–30

Kemmis S (1985) Action research and the politics of reflection. In: Boud D, Keogh R, Walker D (eds) *Reflection: Turning experience into learning*. Kogan Page, London: chap 10

Klein R, Day P, Redmayne S (1996) *Managing Scarcity*. Oxford University Press, Oxford

Kohner N (1994) *Clinical Supervision in Practice: Work from Nursing Development Units*. King's Fund Centre, London

Kolb D (1984) *Experiential Learning: Experience as Source of Learning and Development*. Prentice Hall, New Jersey

Knowles M (1984) *The Adult Learner: A Neglected Species*. Gulf Publishing Co, Houston

Lowry M (1998) Clinical supervision for the development of nursing practice. *Br J Nurs* **7**(9): 553–8

Luft S, Smith M (eds) (1994) *Nursing in General Practice A Foundation Text*. Chapman and Hall, London

Lynch TG, Woelfi NN, Steele DJ, Hanssen CS (1998) Learning style influences student examination performance. *Am J Surg* **176**(1): 62–6

Main A (1985) *Educational Staff Development*. Croom Helm, London

Mairis E (1992) A good example and a lasting impression. *Prof Nurse* **8**(3): 143–6

Malone N (1994) Hydration in the terminally ill patient. *Nurs Standard* **8**(43): 31–6

Mansfield B, Mitchell L (1996) *Towards a Competent Workforce.* Gower Publishing Ltd, London

Marrow CE, Macauley DM, Crumbie A (I997) Promoting reflective practice through structured clinical supervision. *J Nurs Manage* **5**: 77–82

McKinley RK, Fraser RC, van de Vleuten C, Hastings AM (in press) Formative assessment of the consultation performance of medical students in the setting of general practice using a modified version of the Leicester Assessment Package. *Medical Education*

McMahon R, Pearson A (eds) (1991) *Nursing as Therapy.* Chapman and Hall, London

Merrison A (1975) *Report of the Committee of Inquiry into the Regulation of the Medical Profession.* HMSO, London

Mezirow J (1983) A critical theory of adult learning and adult education. *Adult Educ* **32**(1): 3–24

Minghella E, Benson A (1995) Developing reflective practice in mental health nursing through critical incident analysis. *J Adv Nurs* **21**: 205–13

Mitchell A, Cormack M (1998) *The Therapeutic Relationship in Complementary Care.* Churchill Livingstone, Edinburgh

Morgan S (1996) Gods, demons and banshees on the journey to the magic scroll: the use of myth as a framework for reflective practice in nurse education. *Nurse Educ Today* **16**: 144–8

Morris-Thompson P (1999) Nursing and re-engineering. *Nurs Standard* **13**(17): 33–4

Munhall P (1993) Unknowing: Towards another pattern of knowing in nursing. *Nurs Outlook* **41**(3): 125–8

Murphy K, Atkins S (1994) Reflection with a practice-led curriculum. In: Palmer AM, Burns S, Bulman C (eds) (1984) *Reflective Practice in Nursing: The Growth of the Professional Practitioner.* Blackwell Scientific, Oxford

Murray GC, McKenzie K, Kidd GR, Lakhani S, Sinclair B (1998) The five accomplishments: a framework for obtaining customer feedback in a health service community learning disability team. *Br J Learning Disabilities* **26**: 94

O'Brien J (1992) Developing high quality services for people with developmental disabilities. In: Bradly VJ, Bersani HA (eds) (1992) *Quality Assurance for Individuals with Developmental Disabilities.* Paul H Brooks, Baltimore

Palmer A, Burns S, Bulman C (eds) (1994) *Reflective Practice in Nursing: The Growth of the Professional Practitioner.* Blackwell Scientific Publications, Oxford

Pendleton D, Schofield T, Tate P, Havelock P (eds) (1984) *The Consultation: An Approach to Learning and Teaching.* Oxford Medical Publications, Oxford

Preston-Whyte ME, Fraser RC, McKinley RK (1993) Teaching and assessment in the consultation: a workshop for general practice clinical teachers. *Medical Teacher* **15**: 141–6

Powell A (1991) Reflection and the evaluation of experience: pre requisites for therapeutic practice in nursing as therapy. In: McMahon R, Pearson A (1991) *Nursing as Therapy.* Chapman and Hall, London

Rankin S (1996) Disorders of the pregnancy. In: Bennett VR, Brown LK (1996) *Myles Textbook For Midwives.* Churchill Livingstone, London

Ramsden J (1997) Objective analysis of a critical incident. *Nurs Times* **93**(34): 43–5

Royal College of Nursing (1998) Nursing update, Caring together clinical supervision. *Nurs Standard* **12**: 22

Richardson R (1995) Humpty Dumpty: reflection and reflective nursing practice. *J Adv Nurs* **21**: 1044–50

Robbins H, Finley M (1998) *Why Teams Don't Work.* Orion Business Paperbacks, New York

Rogers CR (1967) *On Becoming a Person.* Constable, London

Rogers CR(1969) *Freedom to Learn.* Merril, Ohio

Sandler J (1976) Counter-transference and role-responsiveness. *Int Rev Psychoanal* **3**: 43–7

Schank MJ (1990) Wanted: nurses with critical thinking skills. *J Cont Educa Nurs* **21**(2): 86–9

Schein EH (1987) *Process Consultation Volume II: Lessons for Managers and Consultants.* Addison-Wesley Publishing Co, London

Schön DA (1983) *The Reflective Practitioner; How Professionals Think in Action.* Basic Books, USA

Schön DA (1988) *Educating the Reflective Practitioner.* Jossey-Bass, London

Shen S (1997) China's scientific community denounces superstition and pseudo science. Skeptical briefs 7: 11–15. In: Ullet GA, Hans S, Hans JS (1998) Traditional and evidence based acupuncture. *Southern Medical Journal* **91**(12): 115–1120

Smith EM (1995) *The Nurse Endoscopist. A proposal for the adjustment and development of the nurse's role in endoscopy.* Unpublished Paper, MSc

Smith EM (1999) Developing nurse endoscopy through re-engineering. *Nurs Stand* **13**(18): 35–36

Sweet BR, Tiran D (1997) History and development of the midwifery profession Part 17. In: Sweet BR (1997) *Myles Textbook for Midwives*. Baillière Tindall, London

Teasdale K (1998) Clinical supervision for all. *Prof Nurse* 13(5): 278

Tiran D(1997) Communications and counselling Part 5. In: Sweet BR (1997) *Myles Textbook for Midwives*. Baillière Tindall, London

Todd (1968) *Royal Commission on Medical Education. Report Royal Commission on Medical Education 1965–1968*. HMSO, London

Tolkien JRR (1937) *The Hobbit*. Tinling & Co Ltd, London

Tutton PJM (1996) Psychometric test results associated with high achievement in basic science components of a medical curriculum. *Academic Medicine* 71(2): 181–6

Twinn S, Roberts B, Andrews S (1996) *Community Health Care Nursing Principles for Practice*. Butterworth Heineman, Oxford

United Kingdom Central Council for Nursing, Midwifery and Health Visiting (1992) *Code of Professional Conduct*. UKCC, London

United Kingdom Central Council for Nursing, Midwifery and Health Visiting (1993) *The Council's Position Concerning a Period of Support and Preceptorship. Registrar's Letter.1/1993, Annex one*. UKCC, London

United Kingdom Central Council for Nursing, Midwifery and Health Visiting (1994) *The Future of Professional Practice, The Council's Standards for Education and Practice Following Registration*. UKCC, London.

United Kingdom Central Council for Nursing, Midwifery and Health Visiting (1995) *Standards for Post-Registration, Education and Practice (PREP)*. UKCC, London

United Kingdom Central Council for Nursing, Midwifery and Health Visiting (1996) *Position Statement on Clinical Supervision for Nursing and Health Visiting*. UKCC, London

United Kingdom Central Council for Nursing, Midwifery and Health Visiting (1998) *Midwives Rules and Code of Practice*. UKCC, London

Wilde O (1894) Phrases and philosophies for the use of the young. In: (1987) *The Works of Oscar Wilde*. Galley Press, Leicester

Wilkinson J (1996) Definition of reflective practice: In: Hinchcliffe S (ed) (1996) *Dictionary of Nursing*. 17th edn. Churchill Livingstone, Edinburgh

Wilkinson J (1999) Implementing reflective practice. *Nurs Standard* 13(21): 36–40

Wolfensberger W (1972) *The Principles of Normalisation in Human Services*. National Institute on Mental Health Retardation, Toronto

Wright SG (1989) *Changing Nursing Practice*. Edward Arnold, London